shattered

tragedy on the mountain

shattered

tragedy on the mountain

*Living with traumatic
brain injury and bipolar madness*

Dr. Donna Nicholson
with Gary Nicholson

DNGN Productions LLC
Austin, TX

First Edition
Manufactured in the United States

Information: DNGN Productions LLC
              www.shattered-book.com
              1-512-266-2722

Publisher's Cataloging-in-Publication Data

Nicholson, Donna.
   Shattered : tragedy on the mountain : living with traumatic brain
injury and bipolar madness / Donna Nicholson with Gary Nicholson.
      p. cm.
   ISBN: 978-0-9890249-0-7
   1. Brain—Wounds and injuries—Patients—Family relationships. 2.
Manic-depressive persons—Biography. 3. Brain damage—Patients—Bi-
ography . 4. Adjustment (Psychology)—Popular works.   I. Nicholson,
Gary. II. Title.
RC516 .N53 2013
616.89`5—dc23

                                                        2013903545

THIS BOOK IS DEDICATED TO:

My son. His support helped me through some of the darkest days of my life. His own quest for peace and healing has not been without challenges, yet he has made the journey with courage and commitment.

My husband who suffered greatly in the aftermath of his accident and resulting traumatic brain injury as well as bipolar disorder. I hope he has now found the peace and healing he was not able to find in this life.

Every one of the 30 million people worldwide who deal each day with bipolar disorder. In most cases it has robbed them of their identity and left their families to wonder who the stranger is that has taken their place.

All who suffer from traumatic brain injury as well as their supporters and especially those who, in service to their country, have come home with a TBI. They were wounded on the battlefield protecting our country and now have another battle to wage—but this time the enemy is far less well defined.

The families who offer support to loved ones with these conditions. I have written this book for you because I was one of you, and I know what your path is like.

It is by going down into the abyss that we recover the treasures of life. Where you stumble, there lies your treasure.
Joseph Campbell

The cave you fear to enter holds the treasure you seek.
Joseph Campbell

CONTENTS

PHOTOGRAPHS

NOVEMBER 1999

On a cold, crisp November morning a truck pulling a fifth wheel RV rolls onto the Zuni Indian Reservation in New Mexico. There is no one around for miles and while it has a stark beauty, it is a desolate spot.

The man driving the rig is a fugitive from the law. He is a tormented, lonely soul who has endured all of the misery he can tolerate. He is past trying to deal with the ever-present depression. He has nothing to continue to live for and has lost all that matters to him.

At one time he had it all—successful career, wife, son, beautiful home and ranch. He had brought his life's dreams to reality. That is all gone now and only memories remain as a constant companion, haunting his every moment.

His life as a respected bank president who worked tirelessly in civic and charitable organizations on behalf of the community he served feels as if it was someone else's life, not his. He is living an unbelievably hellish nightmare, facing at least six months in an Arizona prison. He has nothing left to live for and no way out.

The man stops the truck. He reaches across to the passenger seat, picks up his .45, and puts it under his chin. As the sun rises at his back, the light reflects off the gun's barrel like a sunburst. Tears stream down his face, his hands shake, but he knows this time it is for real. There is no going back. The man's trigger finger begins to pull back and his last thoughts are of the life he has lost, what he had been, and what he has become.

AUTHOR'S NOTE

This is the true story of my husband's freakish and shattering accident that forever changed his life, our son's and mine. The events, conversations and details are as accurate as possible. I used my personal journals as well my son's memory and mine of this tragic time in our lives to write the book.

In order to protect the privacy of the individuals who were part of this incredible story I have changed the names of those persons, as well as the small Texas town where we lived at the time of the accident. In some cases I have purposely avoided providing the names of people and places, instead utilizing titles, personal pronouns or descriptions in order to protect certain individuals and organizations.

I have used my real name, my son's and my husband's as well as the real location of Houston, Birmingham and Colorado Springs, which are central to the story.

shattered

INTRODUCTION

Shattered is the story of a man who had it all: a successful career as a bank president, a loving family, and a beautiful sprawling ranch nestled among the rolling hills and tall pine trees of East Texas, a region of the state characterized by its sparking lakes, world-class fishing and hunting, and black gold buried deep within its soil.

The man was a nationally recognized bank president who had finally realized his life-long dream professionally and personally. He was at the top of his game and in the prime of his life. Yet, in mere minutes this idyllic life was shattered beyond repair. A life-altering horse riding accident in the Weminuche Wilderness of Colorado, known for its dangerous and rugged beauty, left the man with major physical injuries and a traumatic brain injury, which triggered a debilitating mental illness.

The man, his wife and son began the unbelievable journey many families have been forced to take when dealing with mental illness. This is the story of John Larkin Nicholson's descent into the depths of hell that is bipolar disorder, schizophrenia and paranoia and how he lost everything, including his family. This is the story of a journey into the world of illusion and delusion that forever changed his circumstances and tossed John and his family into unimaginable and unendurable pain.

This is a gut-wrenching story as John's family comes to understand how this mental illness steals his identity and leaves a stranger in his place. However, this story is not without hope. It is the story of a wife and a son who struggled to understand why and how through a personal journey to discover the answer, they found healing and peace along the way. This is a story for all who have ever had reason to ask why, and though searching, have yet to find the answer to this question, and who thus have yet to heal.

This story will speak to the hearts and minds of those who are dealing with the results of traumatic brain Injury and bipolar disorder or who are in a relationship of family, marriage or parenting where there is any kind of mental illness. It is insidious. It is a thief and it devastates. Yet, as we see a new willingness on the part of celebrities who are experiencing mental illness to come forward and give it a recognizable face, there is added hope that spouses, children and parents everywhere will find the healing and peace that John's family found.

Prologue
How It Began

In October of 1967, I saw my husband for the very first time. I was attending a meeting of the Harris County Young Republicans' Club in Houston, Texas. If you'd told me then he would be my husband in 13 months, I would have said you were crazy. If you'd told me he would eventually break my heart beyond repair and leave a gaping hole in my life, I would have run faster than I initially did. I was on the run anyway when I first laid eyes on my future husband, John Nicholson, because I'd already had my young heart broken by a man and found it so distasteful that I was willing to do almost anything to keep it from happening again. That early experience left me untrusting of all males and I'd vowed never again to give my heart away.

It didn't take a psychiatrist to figure out the reason behind my pattern of actions when a man asked me out and we got to my door at the end of our date. I was accustomed to saying, "I want you to know that I didn't have a good time, and that is my fault not yours. So, if you are thinking of calling me again, please don't." Invariably they would call again, and I'd point out that I had asked them not to, so why were they calling? Their answers all ran along the lines of, "I just thought you were trying to play hard to get." To which I always replied, "I am not playing. I am not hard to get. I am impossible to get." All these years later, with the insight, maturity and distance that time gives you, I cannot believe I went to such lengths. Actually being rude and unkind, for that is not my nature, just to keep someone from getting close enough to hurt me again.

That was my pattern. So I had just one thought when everyone was leaving after the Young Republicans' meeting and I looked up and saw John, the tall, very handsome and confident president of the club, walking toward me with a determined look in his eyes. *Well, here comes trouble on two legs.* I had no intention of engaging with any man who was so obviously trouble. I turned quickly in the opposite direction and went right through the door marked exit. I was beyond grateful for that exit and congratulated myself all the way home for so cleverly averting a potential problem. My heart was safe.

I wouldn't see John for another eight months, during which time I didn't give him a single conscious thought. Though I didn't intend to ever return to any kind of gathering of the Young Republicans' Club, in June of 1968 a friend who didn't want to go alone dragged me to one of their parties kicking and screaming. While I could appreciate that she didn't want to go alone, my mind was made up. I wasn't going, period. No way, no how. I don't like large parties and it occurred to me somewhere in the recesses of my mind that "troublesome man" just might be there. However, after my friend masterfully guilted me I finally gave in with a promise from her that we wouldn't stay long.

As we walked through the door of the party, the first person I saw was John. The look in his eye told me I wouldn't get off free this time because he intended to meet me. He was standing just beside the reception table and once I'd signed in he leaned down, noted my name and said, "Hello Donna. I'm John Nicholson." I politely returned the greeting, and moved into the party with my friend . As the party cranked up I could hear and see him using his "line" on the many women who congregated around him. I told my friend his line was so lame that I was beginning to wonder what was wrong with the women in Houston as they seemed to be taking it all in. Still, we circulated around the room, met some people and got some drinks. Soon, hoping to make a clean getaway, I suggested that we leave, reminding her she'd promised we wouldn't stay long. She'd just asked for a few more minutes when I realized John was approaching. There went my clean getaway.

He began with the same line he'd proudly and successfully been using with all of the other ladies. I listened quietly, biting my tongue. When he stopped to take a breath I very nicely said, "I've known people who kissed the Blarney Stone but I just never met anyone who swallowed the entire rock before." That said, I found my friend and we left. Poor thing, she had to listen to me rant all the way home about how shallow his approach was, and how gullible those girls were who were all over him batting their eyes and taking it all in. Once we got back to our apartment house and went our separate ways I put it out of my mind and gave the encounter no more thought.

Monday morning some three days after the party my phone rang. It was John. When he said, "Donna, this is John," I replied sincerely, "John who?" I really didn't know who it was. There was a frustrated silence on his end before he said through gritted teeth, "John Nicholson." I replied, "Oh yes, the guy who swallowed the Blarney Stone. How are you?" At that he laughed, and we chatted for a few minutes before he asked if I'd have a drink with him that evening. My first instinct was to say no. I'd known from the first time I saw him that he would give me a run for my money and I just didn't want to take the chance. However, I quickly reasoned that I was only risking one drink, during which I would tell him what I had told all the others—not to call me again—and then I could put him behind me. So, I said yes and we agreed on the time he'd pick me up.

I had a houseguest who had been with me for several months. She was an old and dear friend, who had known me since we were children. Sue probably knew me better than anyone else. She had already commented on my usual *modus operandi* with men, pointing out it wasn't a healthy approach to life. When I told her I was going to have one drink with John and tell him what I told all of the others, she said, "You know Donna, I'm just waiting for the one man who will get under your skin again. You always get under theirs, but you don't let them get close enough to get under yours." That gave me pause. Somewhere in my mind I knew she was right, and that thought disturbed me.

John arrived on time, and off we went. As we were talking over our drinks I waited for the right moment to let him know this would be our one and only date. When I told him, he looked surprised and asked why. I replied that I could tell what kind of person he was. He was very amused, and asked what kind. I told him he was the love them and leave them type and he was not going to do either one of those things to me. John threw back his head and laughed. This was not the response I usually got when I took command of the situation. He looked me straight in the eye, not backing down an inch, and said, "I tell you what. If, two months from now we are still dating, and I am sure we will be, and I have proven to you that I'm not what you think I am, then you owe me a dinner of my choice at a restaurant of my choice in Houston." All I could think was, "What arrogance!" I told him that, though I was not a gambler, even I could recognize a sure thing when I saw it, and there was no way we would be dating again—let alone for two months. He just laughed, and looked as if he couldn't wait to take the challenge.

We left and drove back to my apartment and John walked me to my door. What happened next proved to be one of those pivot points in life. John said "Donna, I don't know who hurt you but he did one hell of a good job because you're pushing me away as fast as you can, and I believe I may just be the best thing that's ever happened to you." With that he turned around and walked down the steps. At the bottom he turned to face me and said, grinning broadly, "Lady, I am just going to marry the hell out of you."

I was stunned. I'd been in control without challenge from the men I'd dated for so long I'd forgotten what it was not to get the last word. I went from stunned to furious as I turned, told him to drop dead, opened the door and then slammed it with all my might. Sue was sitting on the coach reading and jumped as I slammed the door. I told her what had happened, pacing and ranting for about an hour. When I stopped I realized she was smiling, which didn't seem appropriate. She said, "Well, well. I think John Nicholson just got under your skin good and proper." I denied it and stomped off to my room.

It was unsettling that John knew me so well in such a short time. He waited three days to call me again, somehow knowing I would need time and space before I would open up even just a little bit. During those three days I calmed down and began to think about what he and Sue had said to me. I didn't like the picture it painted of who I had become. In that moment, the protective shell I had built that no one seemed able to penetrate began to crack.

When John finally called, he asked, "Are you still mad at me?" When I said I wasn't, his response was, "Great. I'll pick you up Saturday at 10. We're going sailing on Galveston Bay with my bank president and other friends."

Two months later I took him to dinner at the restaurant of his choice so he could collect on his winning bet. Those were the first steps toward our eventual marriage on November 23, 1968 in the Second Baptist Church of Houston. There, in front of our families, dearest friends, members of the Texas political scene and my fifth grade students, John and I made our promises to each other. Promises that proved to be critical as our life together unfolded.

So began our journey. Looking back, I realize that with our marriage I began moving toward the eventual loss of John. I had tried so hard to protect my heart after it was broken the first time, yet, I finally took the risk and opened it to John. Then, after years of my heart healing, having John taken from me hit me with far more power than I had ever experienced. It broke my heart all over again, and it almost broke all of me.

We'd been married 12 years when our lives took a decided shift. During that time, we learned a lot about each other. We learned we were well matched. We both needed a partner who would challenge our minds, set reasonable boundaries, have mutual respect and who had similar personal as well as professional goals. We laughed a lot, and traveled to wonderful and exciting places. There were also some very serious times where we weren't sure we could go the distance. That was when we learned that love is both a strong and a powerful bond and not easily broken if you want a relationship to work. We did, so we worked hard and after twelve years had reached a point of ever-deepening love and comfort with each other. We'd weathered the disappointment of learning I might not be able to conceive the child we so badly wanted. Despairing, we went through all the infertility hoops and loops with a team of Houston's finest fertility experts.

Then came the day when, after so much disappointment including us crying together many times when nothing seemed to work, I returned from a visit with the doctor and called John at the bank with the news that we had finally "caught" a baby. He was over the moon, and we celebrated royally that evening with dinner at one of our favorite restaurants near Rice University. My pregnancy was difficult, and I think we both knew we would not be able to have more than this one child. Because of that, when our longed-for healthy child arrived on July 28, 1971 weighing almost eight pounds, he was all the more precious. Neither John nor I had been around babies growing up so while we knew which end the diapers went on that was about it. We struggled and learned together.

John was calmer with our son Gary than I was. He knew Gary wasn't likely to break and worked hard to convince me of that. I realized just how calm and laid back John was with Gary the first time I left him in John's care. It was Sunday, and John's beloved Houston Oilers were playing. I reminded him he couldn't forget to watch Gary and change his diapers, and that I wouldn't be gone long. He said he could handle it and waved me out the door. I came home a few hours later to find Gary playing in the fenced back yard stark naked. When I questioned John he calmly replied, "Well, once he needed to be changed, it just seemed more efficient to take his diaper off and hose him down with the garden hose as necessary." He and Gary both loved that. They were great buddies during those years and John's pride in his son was immense.

Yet, though we did not know it at the time, the dark cloud of fate was beginning to form. When I married John he had told me the story of his mother's mental illness. After she miscarried twins, something went horribly wrong. She began to manifest the markers for manic depression. When John was born she was beginning her downward spiral but it wasn't yet as obvious as it would become. Then in his early twenties she went on an over-the-top buying spree while in a manic episode. The family first became aware she had spent thousands of dollars when her purchases, including a grand piano, were being delivered to the house. John was the one who eventually had to commit her, which haunted him forever. It also gave him a life-long fear and distaste for hospitals in general and mental hospitals in particular.

At the time John's mother was committed, lithium was not used to treat manic depression. The preferred method was shock treatment, to render the patient docile. Mrs. Nicholson endured a series of those brutal treatments and came home a broken individual. John never forgave himself for that and did not talk about it to me again because it was just too painful. At the time he told me his story, I'd no idea that I too would experience the pain and guilt of committing someone you love to a mental hospital.

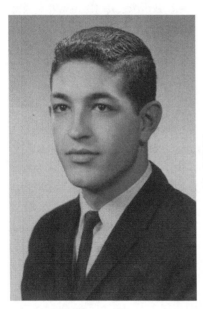

John as he looked when Donna
first saw him at the Harris county
Young Republicans Club in
Houston, TX, October 1967

John as a United States
Marine 1962–66

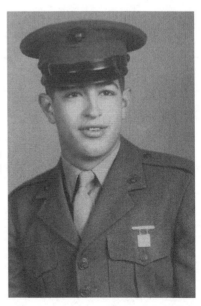

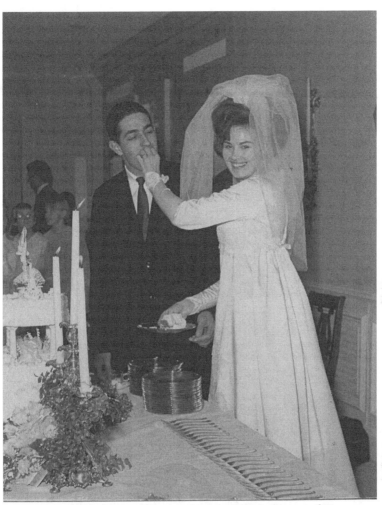

John Nicholson and Donna Marshall Nicholson on their
wedding day, November 23, 1968, Houston, TX

Nicholson-Marshall

Miss Donna Kay Marshall, daughter of Mr and Mrs O. R.
Marshall of Boca Raton, Fla, wed to John L. Nicholson Jr,
son of Mr and Mrs John L. Nicholson, 3805 Tennyson, on Nov
23 in the Second Baptist Church.

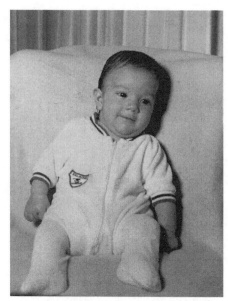

Gary John Nicholson, born July 28,
1971, Methodist Hospital, Houston, TX

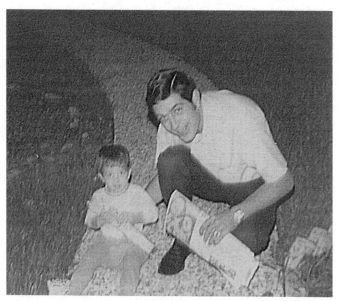

Gary and John (Gary age 2)

PART ONE

THE JOURNEY BEGINS

1
Moving

The summer of 1990 changed all of our lives forever. Neither Gary nor I could have predicted a decade earlier that in ten short years we would be facing the most devastating situation imaginable, and that it would tear our family completely apart bringing such enormous pain it was hard to bear. The contrast between the decade of the '80s and the start of the '90s in our lives is stark. It is hard to imagine such contrast but we know it is true because we lived through every excruciating moment of it.

However, in 1980 there was no shadow to predict what was to come. I came to think of the period from 1980–1990 as the "Life is Good" years. In fact, they weren't just good they were great.

By 1978 my husband John had climbed the managerial ladder of a large bank in Houston. John had served his time as a personal loan officer as well as a commercial loan officer and was ready to take his place as a bank president. That opportunity came when he was hired by a bank about an hour north of Houston in a lakeside community. When we moved, our son Gary and I became the family commuters. Gary, now a first grader, commuted with me since he was a student in the school where I was the principal. Those were wonderful times for Gary and me. During our daily commute we talked, sang songs, and I answered the many questions of his sharp and ever-curious mind. The miles just fell away.

As was John's style, he immediately became deeply involved in this small community, noting the many services which were lacking, and making plans to fill those needs through civic leadership. One gaping and critical need he saw immediately was the lack of medical services within reasonable driving distance. He set about creating an organization devoted to recruiting a doctor. Before John left the community, that one doctor had grown to a full-service clinic with an entire team of doctors and nurses. He was just as instrumental in growing the bank and giving it a high profile within the county. The deposits of the bank grew exponentially and his directors were pleased.

After two years John had made quite an impact on this resort area and it simply was not the same place it had been. Due to his leadership, the small community now had many of the amenities that people in large towns take for granted. Stopping to take inventory, John realized he had done all he thought he could for the community and the bank. He was also becoming unhappy with the constant interference of the bank's major stockholder. That interference often put him in a position where the tightly-held principles of banking which he believed in deeply were at risk. I knew it was just a matter of time until he would no longer be able to tolerate this and would seek a position in another bank.

That happened in early 1980, when John saw an opportunity in the small East Texas town of Jackson. This job would give him the chance to start a new bank and at the same time hold a large share of the bank's stock. He jumped at it. Although I didn't want to leave my job as principal of a new school in a wonderful school district in Houston, I knew I would just have to adjust. John accepted the position of President and CEO of the Independent State Bank in December 1980. When he accepted his new position, the bank was just an FDIC application forming a stack of paper about four feet high, a card table and John's briefcase. Yet in a short time John would make this bank a leader in the industry.

We moved in early December. As I drove out of my school's parking lot for the last time with a sense of loss, great trepidation and many questions, I wondered what this new adventure would bring us as a family.

With all of our things packed, we made the four-hour trip north from Houston to Jackson and settled into a rental house on the outskirts of town. I was almost finished with my doctorate at the University of Houston and had every intention of finishing my degree, which meant I would commute back and forth between Jackson and Houston for a three-day a week stay until I finished. Gary would be enrolled in the elementary school and his life as a third-grader in a new town would begin. Neither John nor I were worried about him because he made friends easily and was a good student.

Our lives quickly settled into a steady but busy pattern of John working long hours to get the bank ready to open, Gary adjusting to a new school and me commuting to Houston. On the days I was in Jackson, I helped John get the bank ready by doing business development for new customers. I even agreed to play bingo with the well-to-do, lovely blue-haired southern ladies of Jackson. I didn't like bingo but I did like them, and they not only opened accounts in the new bank but also got their friends to do the same.

When the bank officially opened its door in the summer of 1981 it was already a huge success due to John's business development strategy. It was giving the other two banks in town a run for their money and John was in his element. He was moving at a very fast pace, getting involved immediately in the community as he had done before. He volunteered for most of the critical committees in town and began to make a difference in a short time. As a family we were happy, exploring the beauty of East Texas and generally making a wonderful transition to this new phase of our lives.

By the end of that summer John and I began to discuss building a home and started looking for property. As a young kid he'd dreamed of living on a ranch where he could raise horses and cattle, so we began talking about fulfilling his dream. I was by no means a country girl but as my dad had always said, "Donna would be happy living on a ranch because of the animals but it would need to be located at 'Fifth and Broadway.'" So my only stipulation in searching for the right piece of property on which to build our home was that it couldn't be far from the bright lights of a city.

2
Dreams Do Come True

As busy as John was with the new bank, he bought drafting materials and began sketching our new home and ranch. It seemed to act as a great stress reliever for him. We spent many evenings discussing the project. Most of the time we agreed on the style of house, but sometimes we disagreed so much we just had to agree to disagree and put the plans away for a while. However, we continued to go on property searches every weekend. John and I also spent time many evenings over a glass of wine discussing the culture shock I was experiencing.

East Texas, while beautiful, was not ready for women to be treated as equals to men in leadership positions and I was having a difficult time with that. I missed my role as a principal and, as I saw it, my prospects in Jackson were grim at best. John always assured me that great opportunities would come to me in my new environment even though it looked hopeless at the moment. He said I would make a great impact on the schools in the area. I couldn't see it. I felt just like Alice in Wonderland when she fell down the rabbit hole. Totally disoriented. But John had always been my mentor and was the one who supported my movement from the role of teacher to that of a school administrator. He saw my talent immediately and had urged me to take the first step to grow into the leader he saw within me. Initially he'd had far more faith in me than I did in myself. In East Texas it was the same story. John never wavered in his belief in me. A couple of years later he was able to tease me and say, "I told you so!"

In terms of females in Jackson's school administration there were two, and both of them were born and raised there—the ultimate insiders, which in a small community is huge. One of them was Gary's elementary principal, who was wonderful. The other was an assistant principal at the high school who was very obviously not treated as an equal by the male administrators in the school.

As we moved into the summer of 1982 John had completed the permanent building for the bank and business was booming. By that fall I had finished all of my remaining course work at the university and was only on the campus two days a week working on my dissertation. That was a relief to all of us. Gary was now a fourth grader and continued to do well. John was enjoying the challenge he had sought in his professional life and had a board of directors that were very supportive without micromanaging.

In early October the one female director of John's bank, who was also the only female on the board of education, approached me to ask if I would apply for the position of assistant principal at the high school, which had just been opened up due to the transfer of one of the male assistant principals. The job was assistant principal for discipline. I laughed and pointed out to her that I didn't think the high school principal or superintendent would be too happy to have an application from a female, especially one who was not from Jackson. While she agreed, she told me the students really needed someone who would approach discipline in a constructive manner and also be their advocate.

When I told John he was delighted, and told me to go for it. I thought it would take a miracle on a level with the Immaculate Conception to be hired in the open position. Not only was I an outsider from the big city of Houston, but I was also a female and would only be available three days a week. "It will never happen," I said. John argued back.

"It's time for a change in Jackson and you are just the one to deliver it, Donna." Ever my mentor and cheerleader, he was convinced I would get the job. I had no such conviction.

As the days rolled by John continued to encourage me to apply. I was also getting lobbied to apply by the high school teachers I had met socially. After thinking about it for several days I decided, "No guts, no glory," and delivered my application to each board member and the superintendent. Later I discovered that delivery threw the entire central administration into a quandary. They didn't know quite how to handle my application because I was the wife of one of the bankers in the town, which carried great prestige, but I was a female applicant. They couldn't just ignore me but they already had a man groomed and ready for the position. What were they going to do?

John was delighted that my application had disturbed the status quo. He told me that when I was interviewed, and they could see what they were really dealing with, their dilemma would only grow. He found the whole thing amusing and kept me focused on the prize. I was as apprehensive as he was amused.

I needn't have worried. After my interview, I called John at the bank to tell him how well it had gone, despite my apprehension. He laughed, saying, "I knew you'd throw them a curve ball. Now let's see what they do with it." What they did was hire me, which had everyone in town talking for weeks and asking how it had come to be. I learned later what had happened from my Houston colleagues, who were called during the reference checking. Apparently I had gotten the job because, as hard as the administration tried to find someone I had worked with who would tell them just one negative thing that they could use to take me out of consideration, they couldn't. They found just the opposite, so I was hired.

John took me to dinner in a neighboring town to celebrate my new job and the major triumph it represented. He chose a popular restaurant and club on the top floor of a high-rise office building for this celebratory dinner. We had almost a 360-degree view of the city with its sparkling lights below. During the evening we leisurely talked about our move and what a positive experience it was proving to be for all of us. We chatted about my new job, his new bank and plans for our new home. John told me how proud he was of me and how much he loved me. I wanted to just freeze the moment. *This is so perfect.* I was almost overwhelmingly grateful at that moment. In the years to come, I would have cause to remember this time and reflect on its perfection. As we celebrated that night, I had no way of knowing that in a few short years all of it would be only a painful memory of a life lost.

3
Living the Good Life

By 1983 John was leading the way as a banker in the state. He'd positioned his bank to survive the devastating crash of the oil and gas industry, which was just beginning to wreak its havoc across Texas. The failure in oil and gas also brought the commercial real estate market crashing down. Propelled by the savings and loan collapse, Texas banks were sucked into a downward spiral from which many of them never recovered. John's bank prospered in spite of this turmoil. He was not only profitable but was also innovating. He was the first to offer branch banking in the state soon after the law permitting it was passed by the Texas legislature. That was quite a coup, and testament to his ability to sense future trends in banking and move quickly yet prudently to take advantage of opportunities before his competition was even aware. He received national recognition for that innovation. John's bank was also in the top 3% of banks their size in the country for performance. Astounding in a climate of enormous economic crisis.

During that year we finally located the property where we would build our home and establish the ranch John had dreamed of for so long. It was fifty-five acres of prime pasture land and best of all for me it was only a mile from the town. The design for the house we had both agreed on by this time was a two-story built into a hill, surrounded on three sides on the bottom floor by earth, and with floor-to-ceiling glass on the entire south-side of the house. Building it into a hill was part of John's design for a passive solar home. He was thinking green long before that became a way of thinking in the world.

There was a perfect hill on the property the right size to position this unique home. The property already had a barn and some fencing as well as three ponds, which we later stocked with fish. It had great rolling expanses of green pastures interspersed with stately oaks and tall pine trees. The beauty just took your breath away. It was as if this piece of property had been waiting just for the three of us to live there. In December of 1984 we moved into our new home and ranch.

John found time from his very busy professional life to erect new fences on the property, clear brush, build a second barn and buy cows at the local sale barn. Gary and I often went with him to the sale barn where we also purchased several quarter horses. It was great fun. John had started Gary on a horse as a young child in Houston so he could get used to the feel of a horse, never fear one and love them as John did. He taught Gary how to ride and how to treat horses.

It was also about this time John got Gary involved in the raising of show steers as part of 4H and FFA. John saw to it that the bank had a high profile as a sponsor of the annual youth project show, which is the heart of small ranching and farming communities in Texas. He supported the youngsters who raised show steers, prize pigs, goats, lambs, chickens and all manner of other farm animals. John always attended the annual auction where these kids would show their animals and sell them to the highest bidder. And his bank was often the highest bidder. Gary was one of the kids who showed and sold their animals, and had a nice collection of Certificates of Deposit in John's bank for the three years he participated. It was truly a joyful life for all of us.

In the early summer of 1985 I stood on the second-floor balcony, which ran the entire length of the house, and breathed in the spectacular view of the pastures. They had just been mowed on this particular day and the hay had been baled. The big round bales lay drying in the pasture with the smell almost wonderfully overwhelming. In the lower pasture the horses and cows were grazing contentedly. I had a feeling of peace followed immediately by one of gratitude for my blessings. Once again I wanted to freeze the moment. It was just so incredibly perfect.

The next three years were a busy whirl of John continuing to grow the bank, me succeeding at the high school beyond my dreams, receiving my doctorate, moving into a regional administrative job and then on to an assistant superintendency in a nearby town. Gary was moving toward graduation from high school and all of us were benefiting from the prosperity we were blessed to have. Each day we fell more in love with the ranch and our way of life, busy as it was.

My way of dealing with the stress of my administrative job was to come home, change clothes, go down to the barn, saddle my horse and ride for over an hour. It just didn't get any better—unless John was able to ride with me. Then we would ride the ranch, checking fence lines and moving the cows from one pasture to another, laughing and teasing each other as we rode. On weekends he worked mending fences. Our favorite time was hanging out at the barn, especially on rainy days, grooming the horses and cleaning the saddles.

During the three-year period from 1985 to 1988 there were many newspaper articles featuring our unique home, which won an architectural award. There were many articles chronicling John's work as a banker and his many innovations as well as the bank's prosperity. There were also newspaper articles about my work. John was producing commercials for the bank and was featured in them on horseback on our ranch. He was at his creative best. All of our dreams were coming true.

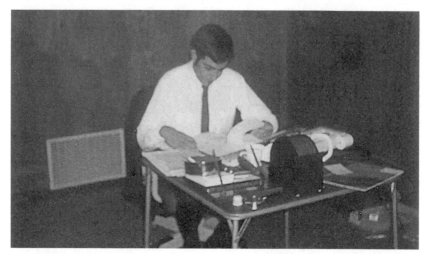

John as president and CEO of the new bank started out in a rented space with only a card table, his brief case and a voluminous FDIC application.

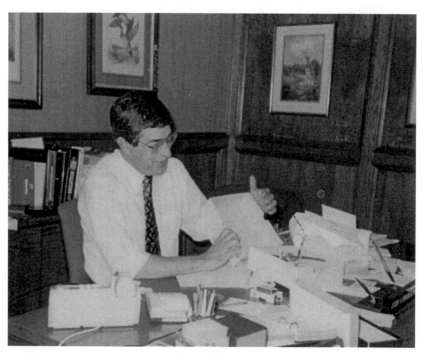

John after the permanent bank building was complete in his new office.

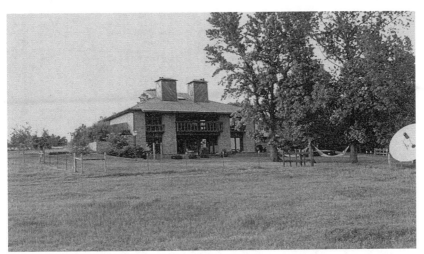

Our dream home and ranch becomes a reality.

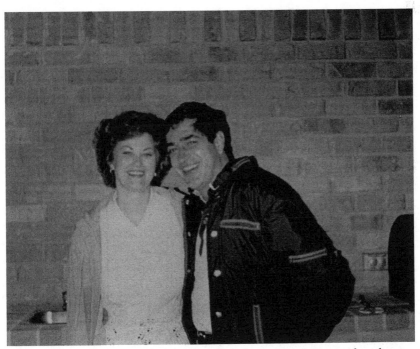

John and Donna on the deck where they often enjoyed wine and nachos.

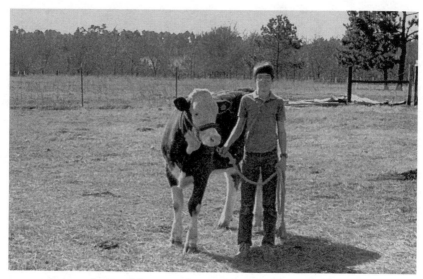

Gary and one of the steers he raised for the youth project show.

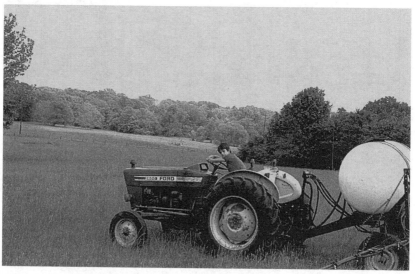

John taught Gary to drive the tractor at an early age.

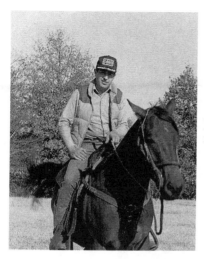

John riding on the
ranch on a winter day.

John taught Gary to ride almost
before he could walk. Gary rides
his horse on our Texas ranch.

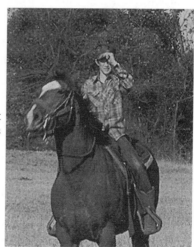

4
The First Two Horse-Packing Trips

In 1988, as we reached the point where our dreams had come true both individually and as a family, John began to show signs of restlessness. He'd started the bank in Jackson in 1981, and seven years later, he had it running smoothly and profitably. However, he seemed to be craving another challenge. Given the state of the Texas economy at the time, the bank shouldn't have been prospering. Many of its competitors were in dire straits. But John was an excellent banker who knew what he was doing. His directors were very pleased and gave him little problem running the bank. He had what he had worked so hard for.

As time went by, I saw more and more of the signs that he had climbed all of the professional mountains he wanted to with this bank. His restlessness was giving way to boredom.

I saw the first signs as he began to drink more heavily. And where once he and Gary had enjoyed a very close relationship, it was beginning to fracture. I was very direct in my discussions with John about his drinking as well as his seemingly constant fault-finding with Gary. At times he would admit he was drinking too much and putting his relationship with Gary at risk, and at other times it was clear he was in complete denial.

During our evening chats over wine and nachos on the deck I began broaching the subject of his boredom. At first he told me no, my perception was wrong. But I continued to gently prod him until he admitted it. "I just don't see what else I can do with the bank, Donna. I've taken it where I wanted it to go."

"Why don't you look for another bank to start or straighten out? There are plenty of those around," I suggested. He said that would probably require a move. "I hate to uproot your career as well as Gary's schooling, not to mention leave our home and ranch." I quickly assured him that while my first choice would not be to uproot Gary, leave my assistant superintendent's position nor our home and property, I was more than willing to do so if he found the right situation where he would once again feel motivated. I also suspected that as he was approaching the age of 46 and midlife, he was reacting to all of the feelings that go with that. He said he would think about it. I could see that he wasn't yet willing to take the kind of risk I'd suggested, but he was ready to take some kind of risk. I was just waiting for the other shoe to drop, because I knew him well enough to know he was going to do something.

In retrospect I realize that 1988 was the beginning of the end of our wonderful lives. The journey ahead of us is one I'd give almost anything for us not to have taken. Yet, as John's 46th birthday drew nearer and with it that mid-life awareness of time running out, we started down the road of no return. His response to those feelings was to do something that would challenge him mentally and physically. So it was that in the summer of 1988 John and three professional colleagues and friends—Jim, Steve and Bob-- began to talk about taking a horse packing trip. Jim and Steve were John's age and Bob was in his early thirties. The older men all wanted to do something to prove they were not over the hill yet. They decided that a horse packing trip was exactly what they wanted to do. All four loved Colorado and agreed to go there on their first horse packing adventure.

That entire year the guys discussed where in Colorado to go. They did their research and decided to ride the Rainbow Trail in

Salida. It's about 11,000 feet above sea level and is a relatively gentle trail. They all had high stress jobs and knew it would be good for them to go a week in the wild without communication with their businesses. The foursome chose to rent packhorses as well as riding horses that year even though we had horses, reasoning that for their first trip they needed experienced mountain horses. John had as usual done meticulous research to find which outfitters had the best horses in Salida. They had a wonderful trip at the end of June and it was without serious incident.

Riding during the day, stopping to fish the crystal clear lakes in the high mountain meadows along the trail, was a singular experience for all of them. Being able to stop at the end of a tiring but delightful day at a well-chosen camping spot, unloading the cooking gear, grilling a thick steak and eating it in the crisp mountain air was almost indescribable. Being able to drink as much wine and whiskey as they wanted without wifely interference wasn't bad either. They would then hobble the horses and tumble exhausted into their sleeping bags to be awakened the next morning by horses nuzzling them or the sun in their eyes.

They decided on the way home that summer this was an experience well worth repeating. They also decided to ride the Rainbow Trail again. The last part of 1988 and the spring of 1989 was once again spent making plans while resupplying their gear and excitedly reflecting on the wonderful experiences of the past year, hoping to repeat them the coming summer. John was happy, and looking forward to these trips helped mitigate his boredom at work.

In late June of 1989 the guys once again set out for Salida and the Rainbow Trail. They again had a wonderful week without incident, renting the packhorses from the same outfitter but taking our horses to ride this time. They had Skip, Red and our baby, Dynamite. All three horses were past those first few years when everything spooks them and they lack confidence. They were all three sure-footed and pretty laid back, from which I took great comfort. Red was my horse and the only Arabian. The others were quarter horses.

I learned quickly after John caved in to my unmovable intention to own an Arabian and bought Red for me that most if not all western horsemen look unfavorably on any other breeds but quarter horses. They especially look upon Arabians as sissy horses because they carry their tails so high when they run and have a very refined and elegant face. While I saw that as beautiful I was teased unmercifully in my part of Texas for having a 'broke-tail' horse, which was their term for the way Arabians carry their tails. So the guys all teased me as they informed me they were taking Red on the trip but were embarrassed to be seen with him. I took it in stride, warning them that they better take good care of my horse and bring him back in one piece.

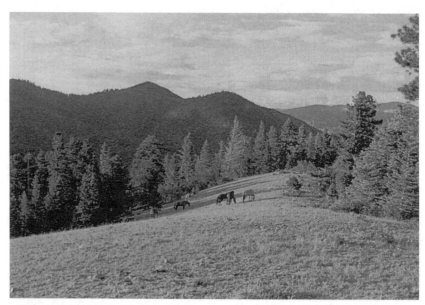

The Rainbow Trail near Salida, CO (1988 and 1989 trips). Resting the horses.

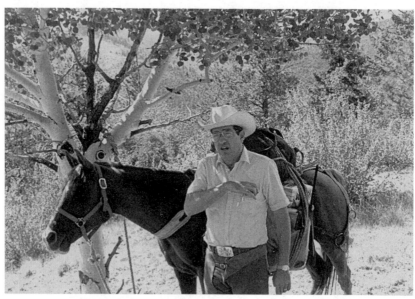

John and Skip taking a break on the Rainbow Trail.

5
A Fateful Decision

While it's difficult to repeat the first-time thrill of a great experience, especially one as enthralling as their 1988 summer on the Rainbow Trail, John and his three friends came close in 1989. Once they knew they had conquered the Rainbow Trail a second time they started talking about where they would go the next summer if they didn't ride the Rainbow Trail. As they discussed this they decided they were ready for a bigger and better adventure. This absolutely appealed to John, the risk-taker, and I imagine he was the one who moved the discussion in that direction.

As they talked things out over the long trip back to East Texas they inched closer and closer to what would become a fateful decision. As the decision hung in the air I imagine the Universe must have held its breath slightly, knowing that this decision would change the course of John's life as well as Gary's and mine forever. They didn't know at that moment just where they would go the next summer, only that the Rainbow Trail was now too tame and they wanted something that would test their mettle. So, throughout the fall of 1989 they researched where they could go that would give them that opportunity.

They finally settled on the Weminuche Wilderness at Wolf Creek Pass, Colorado. The area is particularly rugged and it's not unusual for the police and park rangers to have to rescue hikers, and to find dead horses and their riders. It is very rocky with steep plunging drop-offs. When John told me about the area, I was simply horrified at the prospect of that. I also had a ghastly, intuitive flash of insight about the outcome. But I said nothing until later.

The summer of 1990 only Jim, Steve and John were on the trip. By this time I'd shared my fears with John many times, always ending with a plea not to do this trip, but he couldn't be persuaded. He was beside himself at the prospect of conquering the Weminuche as they had conquered the Rainbow Trail. The contrast between the two locations is enormous and that is just what John was looking for on this third adventure.

Adding to my fear was their decision to use our horses as packhorses, rather than renting experienced ones as they had done the two previous trips. Skip and Dynamite were to be packhorses on the trip and Red would be left behind with me. Having been on the trip in 1989 both Skip and Dynamite were well seasoned but had never been used as packhorses. We would soon come to wonder if that lack of experience in their new role made the defining difference to the trip's outcome.

John was riding a horse he'd bought only a few months prior. Frosty was a two-year-old highly bred quarter horse that had been broken to the saddle but not ridden much. Young horses are spooky and this one particularly so. She was extremely spirited and needed no excuse to go from zero to 60. I was very concerned about John taking her into such a dangerous area for her first trip. I continued to try and talk him out of going, and certainly not to take her if he just had to go. He insisted he could handle everything. I tried to comfort myself with the knowledge that he was an excellent and experienced horseman.

The morning for their third trip to start finally arrived in late June. Just before John left the house to get in his pickup, he hugged and kissed me, once again reassuring me I'd nothing to worry about. I was not reassured. As they left, I watched the convoy of two horse trailers and two pickups move down our long curving driveway with a lump of fear that had lodged in my stomach and would not go away. I could see the dawn beginning to break and the convoy was just a dark silhouette as it crawled toward the highway that would take it to the mountains. I had such a feeling of foreboding. *This adventure will not have a happy ending. Our lives are about to change drastically because of this trip.* Little did I know just how right I was.

The day after the guys left I flew to Atlanta to visit my cousin. It took them about three days to get to Wolf Creek Pass so the day I flew back to Texas was the day they arrived. I continued to have a feeling of foreboding, and on the flight back it just increased. I was convinced that sometime that day I would get a call I did not want to receive.

PART TWO

LIVES ARE SHATTERED

6
The Accident

As I walked in the door of the house from the airport I had that feeling you get when you are just waiting for the other shoe to fall—you know something bad is about to happen but you don't know what. I started unpacking just to have something to keep me occupied but I was so tense I kept dropping things. So I literally jumped like I had been shot when the phone rang about 30 minutes later. I snatched it off the wall with trembling hands and thought I might throw up before I could actually answer it. I wasn't surprised to find Jim on the other end of the line. Before he could say anything except his name, I breathlessly asked if John was still alive. I was certain that whatever I was about to learn would be dire.

He was shocked at my question. As he later explained, he knew there was simply no way I could have known about the accident. Though trying to figure out how I could have known, he quickly answered, "Yes!" but then started beating around the bush about what had happened. I remember telling him with an urgent plea that one of them—he or Steve—needed to just tell me the truth without trying to soften the details, as I knew they would try. I wanted to know exactly what the situation was, no matter how bad it might be. The tone of my voice put him on notice that nothing but the complete truth would satisfy me.

Only at that point did he tell me that John had fallen from his horse and then was run over by the other horses. He said he had been badly hurt—some broken ribs and it appeared something was very wrong with his back. What they could not have known at the time was that his head had also sustained a devastating injury. Jim said it was very apparent that John was in great pain.

They'd taken him to the hospital in Durango where someone had bound his ribs—definitely not the proper protocol for broken ribs. John, being John, had refused to stay in the hospital, and insisted on continuing the trip. His attitude didn't surprise me one bit. As a former Marine he saw himself as tough, and his pride would have made it hard for him to give into pain, even from such severe injuries. However, when they arrived back at Wolf Creek Pass he was coughing up blood and the guys made the decision—despite his protests—that they needed to get back to Texas, and indeed were already headed home. John hadn't wanted me to know what had happened until he could get back and tell me himself. But Jim and Steve made the decision (without John's knowledge) that I needed to know before I saw him because he was so messed up.

When John finally arrived it was a shocking sight. All of my fears prior to the trip had come true and the proof was standing right in front of me. I was numb with disbelief that this person was actually my husband. His face was purple, horribly swollen, and covered with deep cuts and scratches. He was barely walking and stooped over when he did. His forehead not only had gashes which would obviously need stitches but, on closer inspection, I realized there was dirt deeply embedded in the wrinkles. In fact, weeks after the accident we were still removing dirt from his forehead. It was clear that he must have hit the ground with enormous force.

I later learned that the frontal lobe of his brain had been severely injured in the fall, and the injuries were only exacerbated when the horses then ran over his head. The fact that he had not been killed instantly was incredible. How he endured the trip home I will never know, but it's testament to his stubbornness and military training. The enormous pain he was in was clearly reflected in his face. Both Jim and Steve left as soon as they realized that I had every intention of getting him to the doctor immediately, no matter how loudly he might protest. They could see that I was in no mood to let John refuse. But by then John was beyond protesting and I was able to get him into the car with his full cooperation.

It took two years before all the details of the accident were clear. Even now I'm not completely sure we have all of the details, and we likely never will. For a long time John wasn't willing to discuss the accident. He was in and out of the hospital with his physical injuries for about two months and by then it was obvious he had sustained a head injury, which interfered with his ability to clearly remember the sequence of what had happened on that mountain. Both Jim and Steve were greatly shaken by the accident and not anxious to talk about it. Even today, Jim will not talk about it at all.

Piecing together the few details we do have, we believe this is what happened. Once they arrived at Wolf Creek Pass they led the horses out of the trailer and each man packed his packhorse and saddled the horse they were riding. As they set off, the three men were strung out in a line with each rider pulling a packhorse. John was in front with Frosty. Jim was at the back of the line, not realizing he'd packed the coffee pot and lid too close to each other on his packhorse, Dynamite. As Dynamite began to move, the lid rattled loudly against the pot, which frightened the poor horse so badly that he immediately took off, running at top speed. Propelled by sheer instinctive panic he collided with the horse in front, setting off a stampede.

As Frosty in the front of the line realized the other horses were stampeding and on her flank, she raced in a frenzy to get ahead of them, heading for a sheer drop into the canyon below. John struggled to hold her back. He quickly realized there was no way he could hold Frosty back and instinctively pulled her head around—trying desperately to control his runaway horse. She objected mightily to this and responded by bucking him high up into the air.

He landed face first. There were large rocks all over the ground and nothing but their unforgiving jagged points to break his fall. He was knocked unconscious as he came down. By now the other horses couldn't stop. They ran right over him—all five horses, including his own packhorse. In mere seconds it was over, the horses had turned before falling into the canyon and the other two men were kneeling over John's body to determine if he was alive and if so how they could help him.

He was alive but obviously in bad condition. All but one rib was broken, and the bottom two vertebrae in his lower back were crushed. The horses had trampled over his head, leaving him with a closed head injury with a latent response, which was eventually diagnosed as a traumatic brain injury. Much later the doctor explained that football players often are injured in a similar way and the signs of their head injury are not immediately diagnosed or even realized for months. Though the doctors were anxious to know how long John was unconscious neither of the other two men with him knew the answer to that question. They only knew he was unconscious after his fall. I later learned the doctors' interest in this fact was based on their belief that the length of time a person sustaining a traumatic brain injury is unconscious is often an indicator of the severity of the head injury. It is believed that the longer the person is unconscious the greater the brain injury.

How John survived being killed instantly is amazing. We've wondered, but will never know for certain, if the accident could have been prevented if they'd done what they did on their two previous trips and rented experienced packhorses.

Though it made me feel guilty, I came to believe that everyone, especially John, would have been much better off if he'd died on that mountain. For all intents and purposes he did. He just never really came back to us. His physical injures healed, though he had back problems from then on, but he simply never came off of that mountain in any mental condition remotely resembling the person who went up the mountain. That haunted me for the longest time and left me with a deep, hollowed-out feeling. It's beyond difficult when you look at the person you've lived with and loved for so many years and realize that, although the outside looks pretty much the same, the person living inside that physical body is a complete stranger.

There were moments when I felt I couldn't take it. But, I learned very quickly that if I showed any of my emotions it just devastated John. He'd become very insecure and would wring his hands over and over, sometimes pitifully whimpering. So I disciplined myself not to show them, and certainly not to cry where he could see me because it was obvious he was looking to me for his own stability. When I just couldn't hold it together any longer I'd walk down to the barn and play with the barn cats or groom the horses and do my crying there. Animals have a unique way of providing comfort to humans, and they were certainly my comfort then. Sometimes I'd just go outside and sit with the dogs, put my head in their fur, and cry. But after a while I'd learned to hold the emotions in so tightly that I could no longer cry, even when I desperately needed to.

It would be two long months of being in and out of the hospital for treatment of his physical injuries before signs of memory loss as well as completely bizarre behavior became apparent. John was so incredibly intelligent he was able to function, although his reaction time was much slower and he had problems with his short-term memory. The meds he was taking also made him move and talk slower. In the first year after his accident I'd frequently see glimpses of the real John, and I'd silently plead for him to stay. But in a matter of minutes he'd fade back into the stranger he was becoming. As time went by, the real John appeared less and less until he was gone completely.

Most of the time John was aware that he was forgetting things because he'd say to me, "I know you told me something important but I can't remember it." Then he'd become very agitated and often end up in tears. That was particularly difficult for me to deal with because he'd always seen himself as the indestructible John Wayne type: a very independent, hard-charging, get-it-done person who expected a great deal of himself and everyone around him. He was now the complete opposite.

The real John was a gifted leader who was both tough and tender. He was also someone who needed to control. To see him become a person who was needy, clinging and emotional was devastating. He was aware on some level that he was vastly different and that only added to his frustration. I thought it very cruel that he had that awareness. It would have been so much easier for him if he hadn't realized his limitations. However, even though he realized something was amiss, as time went by I understood that he lacked the necessary insight to admit he was mentally ill. Years later I learned that is a very common attribute of bipolar individuals which explains to some degree their resistance to taking their medicine— they don't believe the problem lies with them but with those around them who just don't get it.

John's behavior over the eight years I remained married to him after the accident, along with his bizarre actions, wore me down. I came to the place where I didn't like this stranger, let alone love him anymore.

7
The Aftermath

John was no longer able to go to the bank and work because his back was so injured that he couldn't sit for any period of time without great pain so he was trying to keep up with things by phone. One of his trusted executives, Mary, would also come by to discuss bank affairs, and bring him things to read and sign. But, John was having a difficult time of that, struggling to process things mentally.

Those were devastatingly lonely and scary months for us both. Where once John and I had enjoyed our intimate times, the meds he took left him uninterested and unable to continue that part of our lives. He was aware of his deficit in this area and it caused him great stress. I did my best to assure him he would get better and I was interested in all of him, not just that aspect. He couldn't accept this. He began to believe that I would surely leave him since he was not the person he once was. I am intensely loyal and faithful and he knew that about me, so on a rational level he knew he had nothing to worry about. But that was just the point: he was swiftly becoming less and less rational and more and more paranoid about everything. I reached the point where I simply didn't know what to do to help him through. Finally I came to the conclusion that I couldn't help him and that I just had to accept the situation, support him to the best of my ability and work around it.

Gary graduated high school but told us he wasn't yet ready to go on to college. Instead, in late September of 1990, he left to begin working in Colorado. Prior to his move he was still living at home but, as normal teenagers do, was frequently out with friends (in fact I had encouraged him to spend time with his friends to get away from the gloom of his father's condition) so he didn't see much of the new behavior his father displayed day to day—until the fateful day John had his first real overt display of the effects of his traumatic brain injury.

As John and I were getting up one morning he sat back down on the bed saying, "I feel like something just moved from the back of my head to the front." Then he jumped up and began wringing his hands, frantically repeating, "I have to get out of here!" As he started looking for his car keys I convinced him to let me drive him wherever he wanted to go. We got in the car, but were no more than two miles from home when he started screaming that he had to get out, and began opening the door. I talked him out of that by assuring him we were turning right around and going home. I was terrified.

When we got home I tracked Gary down, then called the doctor and described John's behavior. He immediately said he'd meet us at the local hospital emergency room. John was angry with me for calling the doctor and refused to go. I talked to him for about 30 minutes before I could coax him into the car. The whole journey I was afraid he'd try to get out of the car again while it was moving, but we made it safely. Gary met us at the hospital. Through the years, friends who've heard this story have asked why I didn't ever call someone to help Gary and me when this and other similar incidents occurred. The simple answer is I felt an overwhelming need to protect John's privacy. He was such a private and proud person I knew he'd be devastated if he thought everyone else knew what was happening to him. Plus, I didn't *know* what was really happening.

By the time we reached the hospital, John was hyper, frustrated and again wringing his hands in panic. The doctor met us and got him calmed down, but he kept on wringing his hands and was greatly agitated until the meds took effect. Not long after we arrived, I realized a couple of John's bank directors were there and trying to support all of us. I don't remember how they were notified but I do remember appreciating their presence. When the doctor said he thought that the trauma of being so badly injured physically had caused John's behavior, the bank directors seemed to accept this rationale without much concern, particularly as the doctor made it sound as if this behavior was only temporary, to be expected and it would get better.

Although today this lack of concern and misdiagnosis seems surprising, it must be remembered that in 1990, with Operation Desert Storm and the wars in Iraq and Afghanistan still ahead of us, traumatic brain injury was neither well diagnosed nor the severe consequences well understood. As a result of those wars and the prevalence of head injuries incurred by our troops, doctors now understand so much more about this type of injury.

John's stay in the hospital was short this time. He came home very quiet and dispirited, soon sinking into a deep depression and talking very little. At times I'd find him crying quietly. It hurt me to see him so very broken and to be unable to make him better.

To make matters worse, no one but me was seeing the day-to-day manifestations of John's head injury. Our family doctor was sympathetic but said he just didn't see anything but a man recovering from physical injuries who wasn't accustomed to such limitations. Not surprising that the doctor didn't see what I was seeing because John was an amazing actor during this time. I don't know whether he consciously determined that he would act just as he always had or if it was something else. I do know that he became Dr. Jekyll and Mr. Hyde. He was his pre-accident Mr. Charming, funny and quick-witted once he got out the door of the house. So, when I went to the doctor with him, Mr. Charming went with me, even though minutes before leaving the house he was the very disturbed person he'd become and the one I was trying desperately to describe to the doctor.

The doctor would look at me strangely when I tried to describe John's behavior at home and I expect he was thinking that I was the one who'd lost it. There were many times when I thought I *was* crazy but I knew John's behavior wasn't normal. I was right, as his strange behavior was to escalate in October of that year and by November he'd had his first full-blown manic episode. That culminated in the first of three times over the next eight years that I had him committed to a psychiatric hospital.

When Gary left in September it hit John very hard. He was teary a lot of the time and I knew he missed Gary terribly. He would often look at me with such sadness and ask me how I was coping with Gary being gone. "Aren't you feeling bad?" he'd ask. I'd admit it was hard and that I did feel sad. "But it's a necessary and normal process of Gary growing up," I'd say. "I know he'll be in touch, and he'll come home for holidays." Yet, John's behavior was deteriorating into bizarre phone calls to Gary as well as people we knew across the country. Many of them had no idea what had happened and called back to ask if he was okay. I tried to keep it simple by thanking them for their concern, explaining that he was sick but getting better. If only that had been true.

My nerves and patience were running very thin because I was still working full time as an assistant superintendent and balancing that with my care of John. I'm normally a very compassionate and caring person but I found myself snapping at him, and wanting to tell him to suck it up. That kind of behavior wasn't the norm and I knew it, which filled me with such guilt. I later learned not to be so hard on myself, reminding myself no way was I ever Mother Teresa. In fact I have a very feisty, sassy personality so the wonder is that I didn't snap more often. However, to this day I still inwardly flinch at my frustrated responses, even though they were infrequent and fleeting. Intellectually, I know my behavior was both understandable and forgivable, yet my heart still cringes. I can't erase the look on his face when I treated him that way.

Things rocked on with John manifesting moments of great depression and moments of euphoria, which spawned more bizarre behavior. One evening he told me to be very quiet because the FBI had our house surrounded and bugged. I asked him why they would do that, and he replied, "Because I work for the CIA and they don't like me." I tried to reason with him at first, pointing out that he didn't work for the CIA, the FBI wasn't outside our house, nor was the house bugged. That only made him more argumentative and hyper. I finally just left the room before I made things worse.

On November 11, 1990 John woke up higher than a kite, his speech fast and euphoric. I knew we were headed for something awful, and that it would be something I'd not seen from him before. We'd already invited a couple of friends over for dinner because John convinced me he was feeling better and thought having friends over would be a welcome relief. When they arrived they knew something wasn't quite right. If I'd had any idea what was about to happen I would have called off our dinner party. Never having experienced the aftermath of a traumatic brain injury or bipolar behavior, and still wondering if what I thought I was seeing was my own craziness, I just went with our original plans.

After dinner John started talking about world monetary systems and predicting that one day we wouldn't need money to do business, just smart cards. Remember, these were the days prior to debit cards. I thought nothing of it since our guests were bankers and it seemed an obvious topic of discussion. To prove his point, he said he was going to leave for a few minutes, go down to the corner store to "buy" some things and that he wouldn't take money or credit cards, whereupon he emptied his pockets. (The logic of that escaped not only me but also our dinner guests.)

I started to call the doctor right then, but decided to wait and see what would happen. When John got back he had an armful of junk from the store, which he put on the coffee table, saying, "See, I got all of this without any money or credit cards." The lady who operated the corner store knew him well as he stopped there for coffee every morning. It was no wonder she let him take the items he selected without paying her. She later told me she was so stunned by his very uncharacteristic behavior all she could do was just stare at him, speechless. After making his point that he was able to purchase things without money or a credit card, he said he was going to charter a plane to Las Vegas for all of us. From Vegas, we would all go around the world doing Jesus' work. In a few more breaths he said he *was* Jesus. This was especially bizarre because John was not a religious man and he disliked Las Vegas.

He then bolted to the kitchen phone and called the airport to charter the plane. He knew exactly who to talk to because as bank president he'd chartered planes when we needed to get to Dallas from our small regional airport to connect with flights to conferences. Therefore, when he called the airport that night, chartering a plane wasn't seen as an unusual request. After he'd finished, I simply went to the second line in the house, called the airport and cancelled what he'd booked. The person I spoke to was the same one John had just talked to and he commented that he didn't seem like himself. "Is John okay?" he asked. I thanked him for his concern, but had neither the energy nor inclination to say anything more than, "No, he's not okay."

8
His First Psychiatric Hospital Commitment

My next call was to the doctor. I briefly described John's behavior. "This is the worst I've seen, but it's the same kind of behavior I've tried to describe to you for the past two months although you've never seen it," I told him. "John's so manic, he's going to need something to get him calmed down." The doctor agreed, and said he'd be there as quickly as possible.

I met him at the door, and as John was in another room with our guests he didn't hear us talking. The doctor told me he'd stopped by the county judge's home on the way over to get him to sign a committal form so, with my counter signature, he could put John in the nearest psychiatric hospital. I must have been in shock because what he said just didn't sink in at first. All I said was, "Well, let me get my purse and I'll go with you all to the emergency room." I suppose I was assuming we'd go back to the Jackson hospital where we'd been in September. The doctor gently said, "No, you don't understand Donna. We're not going to the emergency room here in Jackson. We're going to the psychiatric wing of Mercy Hospital."

He explained that by law John had to be taken there by the sheriff, and not just accompanied by him, but in the back of the sheriff's car behind the wire divider. He told me that they could also cuff him if John hadn't responded to the sedative he was about to give him. He made it very clear that I wouldn't be permitted to go with John. As he spoke, the doctor could see that the enormity of the situation was beginning to dawn on me. Very kindly he said, "Donna, this is going to be the hardest thing you've ever been asked to do but we must do it for John." I remember him handing me the committal form and pointing out where I needed to sign. As I reached for the form and prepared to sign it, everything seemed to be happening in slow motion. As I signed, I felt as if I did it from a great distance. I was struggling to process what had been said to me and what I'd just done. (I felt totally disoriented, unable to get my bearings.)

The doctor then gave John a shot of sedative. He didn't resist, partially because he trusted this man but also because the manic episode was starting to wind down on its own. To say I was numb would be an understatement. I hugged John, told him it would be okay and that I couldn't go with him but would see him the next day. I also told him I loved him. Once the door closed behind John and the doctor I stood with my head down for a moment, wondering what in God's name we were going to do to make it through this latest heartbreak. It was then I realized our dinner guests were still there. That simply took my breath away and left me lightheaded, as they had just had a front row seat to John's most humiliating and devastating moment. And two of them worked for him at the bank. I'd no wish to hide John's condition from the staff or board of directors. I did, however, very much want him to be able to deal with his illness with dignity and maintain some control over how he chose to deal with his departure from the bank with his board and staff, when the appropriate time came. It was my intention to help John accept this latest turn of events and create his own way of letting them know he was not well as a result of his accident.

Then it hit me like a ton of bricks: the fact that two bank employees just witnessed John's first manic episode and ultimate committal had removed that possibility in a split second.

They had seen him being taken by the sheriff in the back of his official car to the psychiatric hospital. They had seen me sign the very papers which made that possible. It is a measure of how out of it I was that I had not asked them to leave after I called the doctor earlier in the evening. *Why, oh why, did I not do that?* Now I felt utterly helpless to stop what felt like a giant snowball rolling downhill toward our family. I added the guilt I felt for not handling this latest crisis to my growing stockpile of guilt. My failure to have John's back in this most critical moment left him even more vulnerable than he already was.

If I'd had any doubt that John's banking career was over due to his accident, I now knew it for certain. I also knew how completely this knowledge would knock him to his knees. He'd not even begun to accept that he was mentally ill, and I don't believe he ever really did. It was just too horrendous an idea for him to even look at, let alone accept. His identity was so bound up in his position as the president of the bank that I am certain, to the day he died, he still saw himself as that same banker who went to the bank everyday in his starched white dress shirts and beautiful suits.

That evening of November 11 was to be the first of many times over the next eight years that I would feel completely helpless, utterly devastated and as alone as I have ever been. I am by nature a person not given to being lonely, so I was in new territory. I'll never forget the lost and wounded look in John's eyes when the sheriff took him away. My heart literally hurt for him and what he was going through. I could imagine only too well how lost, confused, hurt and alone he must feel too, yet he wasn't allowed even a single family member to be by his side, to hold his hand, to support him. I heard again in my mind the pain and anguish with which he'd told me early in our life together about the time he'd had to commit his mother. I knew only too well how very much he hated hospitals, and especially mental hospitals. Now I'd also committed someone I loved to a mental hospital. And I understood.

I wasn't allowed to visit John until the next afternoon. By that time he'd found a way to escape from the psychiatric ward, go down the street to the fire department, and somehow steal a fire truck. He was caught driving it very slowly down Main Street. His leadership talents always included his ability to solve problems and be resourceful in the face of huge obstacles. He'd also been a Marine who'd served in Viet Nam. In short, he had many skills, which clearly served him well in trying to escape from that hospital.

I didn't know about the fire truck misadventure when I arrived and was shown to his room. Apparently, after his escape the staff had given him massive doses of Haldol, which I soon learned is a very potent drug although when used in mild doses will calm patients. By the looks of things they'd given John way too much. He was curled up in a fetal position on the bed shaking and sobbing. It stunned me at first and then made me so angry I went tearing out of his room looking for a nurse. When I found one I asked nicely but firmly why they'd given him so much medicine. They patronizingly assured me he was fine. I just wanted to strangle them.

"Call the doctor immediately," I demanded. "Or I will." They tried again to patronize me. I let loose on all of them and moved toward the phone. Seeing I meant business, one of the nurses said she'd call the doctor. He arrived very quickly and went into John's room. What he saw made him as mad as I was, and he demanded to know who'd given this patient such a large dose. After much scurrying, the staff finally began to work on John to correct their negligence.

While they were working, I called our Jackson doctor and told him I wouldn't leave John in that hospital under any circumstance. He said the psychiatric hospital in the largest town in the area, about 45 minutes away, was a much better option and the psychiatrist who would be handling John's case, Dr. McNamara, was one of the best. He called Dr. McNamara and alerted him that I'd be calling in a few minutes. When I called, I was assured they'd take John. I called our family doctor back and told him I'd talked to Dr. McNamara, was convinced he could help John and confirmed the information he'd need for the hospital before we transported him.

That's when he told me he'd have to be transported the same way he'd first arrived—by the sheriff.

Taking a deep breath, I told the doctor to inform the Jackson sheriff there was no way John would be riding to the new hospital all by himself in the back of the car as he had the day before. "I'll be sitting next to him holding his hand the whole way," I said. "And tell the sheriff, if he tries to stop me, I promise I'll throw the worst Southern hissy fit he's ever seen. Right there in the parking lot." The doctor assured me he'd convey my message and doubted there would be any resistance. He was right.

That ride to the new hospital was another of those seminal moments I'll never forget. It was an experience so sad that the sadness settles in your bones. John was still shaking and sobbing, clutching my hand like an eight-year-old. Here was a man who'd been a nationally acclaimed banker and a brilliant individual, reduced through a head injury to a tragic parody of himself. To the day I die that image will be with me.

9
The Hell of Madness

D r. McNamara met us at the new hospital, where the staff asked me to stay in the waiting room and tried to take John away. When he realized we were going to be separated, he began to resist. He didn't want me to leave but Dr. McNamara and I convinced him that I wasn't going anywhere, and would see him in a few minutes. I waited alone for what seemed like an eternity. I was still numb, and remember feeling like this was an out-of-body experience.

Finally, Dr. McNamara came out to talk to me. They were examining John and he wanted to know if he had any negative reactions to medications that I knew of. I explained that he didn't like to take medication and resisted taking even an aspirin. (That likely stemmed from the fact that his sister had been addicted to drugs.) However, I did warn him that on the few occasions when John took meds it didn't take much for his body to over react, citing the recent incident with Haldol as a perfect example.

With that, Dr. McNamara told me to go home. He'd call when he had a diagnosis or any news. I thanked him but said I'd stay. Hours later he confirmed that John had indeed suffered a traumatic brain injury. As a result he was now bipolar disordered, suffering from paranoia and perhaps some schizophrenia. As I hung on his every word, Dr. McNamara explained that bipolar disorder is either hereditary or the result of a trauma. Today some doctors disagree with that and instead believe it is hereditary and think it can be triggered by a traumatic injury if the patient has a proclivity for it. So, it can lie dormant until something like a traumatic brain injury sets it in motion. Even great stress is thought to trigger it.

With my mind racing, and thinking about John's mother and her bipolar disorder I was profoundly confused. I knew I'd never seen any signs that he was bipolar disordered until after his accident. He'd had an expansive personality but within normal parameters. He was extremely responsible and I didn't see huge mood swings typical of bipolar. I had questions—lots of them. If somehow John's bipolar was a result of heredity what implications did that have for our son Gary? Had John inherited the proclivity for bipolar and it had lain dormant until his accident? I knew I needed to find answers to these burning questions.

The most immediate question was, now that we had a diagnosis, how was the doctor going to treat it? Was there a cure? "I'm afraid there's no cure for bipolar disorder, Donna," Dr. McNamara said. He went on to explain that John would be treated with a combination of drugs and psychiatric counseling. "The best we know is how to manage it, not cure it," he told me. Since no two human brains are exactly alike there's no standard dosage of medicine for patients with this disorder because there is no such thing as an "average" brain when it comes to amount given and reaction to medication, explained Dr. McNamara. It would probably be 24 hours at least before they could gauge if the dosage initially given would be workable.

He then insisted there was nothing more I could do so I needed to go home and get some rest. As if I could do that. However, this time I agreed. It was a 45-minute drive, and what a terrible drive it was. It was dark, the road was winding and difficult to negotiate, and my mind was working overtime. Through all of this, I'd never asked, "Why me?" But that night I began asking, "Why?" Although I didn't realize it at the time, I was to become a driven seeker of the answer to that simple question, which in turn provided me with the greatest personal growth I've ever experienced.

I'd cried very little since John walked through the door after his accident. As I mentioned, I was so devastated I couldn't cry and I also understood I needed to stay strong for him. Plus, I've never been much of a crier, preferring instead to use my energy on solutions and moving forward. As I'm a very pragmatic person, that mindset fits me better than crying. Today I understand that crying is healing. It comes from the heart and the soul and while wrenching it eventually leads to peace and acceptance.

However, when I got into the house that night all of the events of the months since the accident closed in on me. I stepped into John's closet, took one of his suits in my arms, and sobbed. I felt so utterly bereft and adrift. I didn't know what to do or how to react because for one of the few times in my life I couldn't control my environment. And it was so out of control. I couldn't make John better. I couldn't turn the clock back to before the accident. Here I was standing in his closet sobbing, so I couldn't even help myself. I also had no idea what to expect when I returned to the hospital the next day. This was without a doubt a full-blown dark night of the soul experience the likes of which I'd never encountered. Again I asked, "Why?"

10
Close To Death

The next morning Dr. McNamara called with stunning news. John had experienced a violent reaction to the medication, was in a coma and I needed to get his affairs in order because they didn't know if he'd make it. Somehow I managed to call Jim and Steve before I raced to the hospital. I don't remember the drive, which I'm sure I made at break neck speed because my heart was beating so hard and I was in a full-blown state of panic.

Jim lived only a few miles from the hospital and came immediately. He tried to get me to go eat something, but I couldn't. Finally he insisted, taking me to a restaurant but I still couldn't eat. He talked a little bit about what had happened in Colorado, and I remember getting some more details about John's accident. Steve, who lived a hard eight hours away in another state, got in his car after hanging up from our call and drove non-stop to the hospital. He was clearly shaken when he arrived. I was so glad to see them both, and we waited together for hours.

Sometime that night, Dr. McNamara came into the waiting room to say that John seemed to be rallying and he was cautiously optimistic about him. In fact, John did improve physically as the days went by. I settled into a routine of going to work, which was forty minutes away in one direction, and then after my day ended driving to visit John, a 45-minute trip in another direction, then driving home 45 minutes in yet another direction. Those were days of both physical exhaustion and mental anguish, as John grew stranger every single day.

His paranoia and delusion were unbelievable. He became convinced that I had him committed because I was actually "shacked up" with a man in our home in Jackson. When one of his customers and his wife, who were very religious, visited him in the hospital John convinced them of this ludicrous story, and that he was an unwilling prisoner of the hospital because I had him committed. The couple called me frequently, begging me do the right and Christian thing by getting John out of the hospital. They also counseled me to get rid of my live-in lover, because I was committing adultery. No matter how much and how hard I explained that the man John was convinced was living with me was part of his paranoid and delusional state, they couldn't hear me. They were on a mission to protect John. I soon realized that, and had it not been so tragic, it would have been something I was grateful for because it meant we were on the same mission.

Then I began receiving letters from John. Much later, I discovered those two caring but misguided customers were mailing them for him. To say the letters were vile and foreign to anything I'd ever experienced from John Nicholson would be one of the great understatements of all time. John had been initially attracted to me for many reasons, not the least of which was my independent, sassy and direct manner. He considered me a challenge he relished, as did I him. He teased me unmercifully but treated me with the greatest respect. We didn't often argue but when we did it was worth buying a ticket to see because it was like watching two lawyers battling it out in court. We engaged with facts, logic and stubbornness born of knowing we were right and the other person wrong. No question about it.

So when I read the first letter I had to sit down because my knees would have buckled otherwise. I was horrified and couldn't believe he'd written such garbage. It was clear that he was no longer the man I knew but was instead living in a hellish, sick world of fantasy. The first letter began, "Dear Whore." He then launched into a rambling narrative about how I'd tricked him for 22 years into thinking I was a lady and someone who'd had no sexual experience before we married. He said I probably couldn't even remember the number of men I had fucked. Yes, he used that word. One sentence said, "You are a god-dammed whore who will lie down with anything." The letter was liberally laced with profanity of the worst kind. He frequently referred to me as "you fucking whore, slut and adulteress."

He railed at me, saying he knew I had him committed so I could shack up with the man I had living in his house. He demanded to know who it was, and then offered several suggestions of who he thought it was. The list was ludicrous, and would only become funny many years after it was written. He had men on his suspect list ranging from the janitor at the bank, to the man who repaired our cars, to the man who lived on our property and took care of the cattle and horses. It was very clear that I'd become John's enemy in his tortured mind. He'd been my best friend and mentor besides being my husband, so this was very difficult to take. I had to keep reminding myself that the "real" John would *never* have spoken to me this way, certainly knew I was a lady in my behavior, had been faithful and loved him very much. In fact, had anyone ever tried to talk to me in this way he would have beaten them to death.

I was so broken after reading this letter that for the first time since the accident I called my pastor. He knew John, and I reasoned he'd help me deal with this and give it the perspective I so badly needed. He did try, but when he read the letter he was speechless and shocked. Clearly this was beyond his scope of experience. He felt as bad as I did when he left. After he was gone, I walked through the house touching the things I loved, things John had given me, things we had bought together looking for comfort and once again asked God, "Why?"

There were six letters in all but I don't know what the other five said. All I did was open them to check the greeting. They all started with variations of "Dear Whore." I didn't read any further and couldn't bear to keep them, so I tore them up and threw them away. That was as close to an act of cleansing as I knew how to get. Once John got home from the hospital and was on meds and calm, he never mentioned the letters, or the man I'd been accused of living with, nor did he treat me as he did in the letters. I once mentioned to him that I'd received his letters, because I suspected he'd no idea he'd written them. He looked blank and said he didn't know what I was talking about.

11
Life in the Hospital

My daily visits to the hospital became torture for me. Sometimes John would refuse to see me. Other times he would rant and rave, accusing me of all manner of things bearing no resemblance to reality but reflecting the content of his letters. About that time, Dr. McNamara began psychiatric sessions with him, initially asking me to attend. The first session found me uncharacteristically quiet in the face of John's accusations and just plain mean behavior toward me. At the end of that session the doctor spoke to me privately, saying, "Donna, my impression of you is that you are a feisty lady. Why are you taking this from John without as much as a word?"

I explained that I was stunned by John's behavior. I told him about the letters. I told him I didn't really know how to react to John as he was now a complete stranger to me. I also said I was afraid that if I really let go on him it would impede his recovery.

The doctor explained that wouldn't happen and it would help get John back to normal if I reacted exactly as I would if he weren't ill. The following sessions were quite different as I refused to put up with his horrible behavior and more than held my own with him. In fact, several times after warning him to back off and that I would leave if he didn't, I did just that. I'm a world-class door slammer when

I'm mad and John had teased me about it all of our married life so I always did my best when leaving the most contentious counseling sessions to slam the door as hard as I could.

It was also about this time that John, ever a leader, organized the other patients in his area to demand music therapy because he'd read that was healing. Since his version of reality was that he was in the hospital because I had him committed so I could do my evil deeds, he never saw himself as a real patient with any problems. John figured since he couldn't get out, he'd become a patient advocate and help those who really were in the hospital for valid reasons. One of his favorite movies was *One Flew Over the Cuckoo's Nest* and I think he fashioned his patient "revolt" for music therapy after that movie.

He also began demanding his right to be released. As the Internet wasn't an option at this time, he had no way to do his own research. Instead, John had gotten the two customers who mailed his letters to me to get him information about the laws regarding commitment and in short order became an expert on his rights and those of the other patients. He wrote letters to the hospital administrator and hospital board members on his and the other patients' behalf. Needless to say, those letters though elegantly written were studies in madness.

He got his two friends who had mailed his letters to me to take and mail all of them. Once I knew that, I had the hospital ban the well-meaning yet totally misguided pair from visiting. John was furious with me, and after that there were days when I simply couldn't visit. After a day or two of my absence he'd get the doctor to call me and ask if I'd come back to see him if he promised to be very nice. Sometimes he was able to keep his promise and some days he wasn't. On those days my visits were very short.

Of course, although John was a huge part of my life, all of this wasn't going on in isolation. I had my very demanding job as an assistant superintendent for a school district and had to remain an accountable, fully present professional in spite of my personal life, which was falling to pieces. My closest professional colleagues knew what I was going through but most people in the district didn't. Those colleagues assured me that if they hadn't known what I was going through they would never have guessed as I just carried on as usual.

The truth of the matter was that I felt so completely broken inside and fragile that I wondered sometimes if I would last another day. I am a very contained and private person where my problems are concerned. It isn't easy for me to share my feelings and this situation was no different. When you are faced with overwhelming experiences, the like of which you never thought you'd ever have to face, it is then that you learn what kind of stuff you're made of—and I've decided that I'm made of tough stuff. I'm not one to take medicine unless I just have to, so it didn't occur to me to ask the doctor to prescribe something to help me sleep and just get through my days. I've always relied on my grit, stubbornness, determination and ability to survive and so that's what I used. If I'd known then what I've since learned, I would have understood that you just can't go through something like this alone. You need a very strong support system of people who love and care about you: people who don't pass judgment, and who are there for the right reasons. There were people like that in my life during all of this and I did lean on them a little from time to time but not as much as I should have done. I would have been so much better off if I'd allowed them to really help me. My burden would have been so much lighter if I had just reached out more often.

John remained in the hospital for a month. He continued to protest being held against his will and continued to write letters to hospital officials demanding to be released. I continued to visit and found him more and more a stranger. At times he was so glad to see me and at other times he was remote and guarded.

I didn't call Gary when this all happened because I didn't want to scare him by sharing what I was going through and I knew being so far away in Durango he would worry without being able to do anything about the situation. John's episode was November 11 so I made the decision to wait until Thanksgiving before sharing the details. He'd be home then and I'd have more definitive answers about his dad's condition. I thought it important to discuss this face to face. I don't know if this was the right decision but it felt right at the time. Since then, Gary's told me how angry he was at being left out, feeling I didn't trust him enough to tell him. In truth, as I explained to him, lack of trust wasn't my issue. All mothers seek first to protect and shelter their children from harm, and that's what I was trying to do. My mistake came in not realizing that, at 18, Gary was no longer a child, and that he deserved to know and be given the chance to work through things with me. I've since apologized. My only consolation is that, faced with situations like this, we make the best decisions we can, but they're not always the right ones.

The holidays arrived and Gary came home. We had Thanksgiving dinner with John and his counselor in the town near the hospital. His counselor had arranged for a pass so we could celebrate as a family. Unfortunately, it was no celebration. It was a somber, uncomfortable time as John was deeply depressed, anxious and jumpy. Gary was greatly affected and drew into himself to where I couldn't reach him, and I knew I needed to understand much more than I did about John's condition so I could help us all cope. Memories of past Thanksgiving celebrations flooded my mind. John had always been a good cook and liked to try out recipes, so he'd always enjoyed experimenting with different ways to prepare and cook our Thanksgiving turkey. Sometimes he hit a home run and other times Gary and I had to try and tell him tactfully it wasn't our favorite. This year was disturbing for both Gary and me because not only was John in no shape to try out one of his recipes for the turkey, we had no idea if he ever would be again.

PART THREE

THE THIEF THAT IS BIPOLAR DISORDER

12
Please Help Me Understand Bipolar

When I met Dr. McNamara for the first time he told me I needed to consider seeing a psychiatrist or psychologist because this was going to be a rough ride for me. I'd no idea then what he was talking about, but I told him I'd give it some consideration. For the first couple of weeks of John's stay in the hospital I resisted following his advice. I felt I'd surely survive it. All I needed to do was just keep putting one foot in front of the other.

However, as time went by, I had more and more questions about John's bipolar disorder as well as the paranoia and schizophrenia he was evidencing. One of my strongest coping mechanisms had always been to learn everything I could about a potential problem, and from there I'd build strategies to deal with it. So that's what I set out to do this time. Despite my best efforts, and to my frustration, I couldn't find any information about bipolar disorder. I did come to understand that this disorder was a closet mental illness—as it still is to a large degree today. Lots of people had it, but no one talked or wrote about it in layman's terms. Finally I asked Dr. McNamara to recommend a psychiatrist I could talk to. I had one session with his colleague where I got to ask all of my questions, but there were very few answers. And, as I've now realized through my continued research over the years, some of the answers I got then just weren't correct, which I attribute to the lack of knowledge or understanding of this disorder in 1990.

Back then, I simply wanted to know what to expect, and what he could give me to read that would help me understand what John was going through. I wanted to know what the long-term prognosis was, and I wanted to know how I could be of the greatest help to John. The doctor basically told me there were no books, articles or anything else he could recommend on these disorders. "There are only medical journals, Mrs. Nicholson, and I doubt those will be of any help to you," he told me. I was disheartened, but one thing resonated. "John will be better with you than without you," he said. "But you'll have to decide at what point that's not true for you. In most cases like yours, the caregiver spouse stays between two and three years with the bipolar spouse." I stayed for eight.

My next question was the critical one: do bipolar disordered people get violent. His maddening answer was that some do, and some don't. I told the doctor, I loved my husband, and on the 23rd day of November 1968 had stood next to him in the sight of God, promising to stay with him in sickness and in health—which I fully intended to do. "However, if he ever showed me that he was going to be violent that would be a complete deal breaker," I said. "I'll walk away and not look back." Sadly, that day did eventually arrive.

It was to be five years before a book answering more of my questions would appear. In 1995 *An Unquiet Mind* was published by Dr. Kay Redfield Jameson, a psychiatrist on the faculty of Johns Hopkins University, who is bipolar disordered. That was the first time I truly understood why John did what he did and, more importantly, why he wouldn't take his medicine. Dr. Jameson wrote that the manic loop of the bipolar disorder was addictive because the manic high was like nothing in this world. She even called it the "Rings of Saturn," because it was so out of this world. Unlike cocaine or heroin, the bipolar manic highs get better and better each time. If you're on a manic high it feels like money is in inexhaustible supply, there's nothing that can't be overcome, and your creativity and intelligence is at a level well beyond the norm. Why would anyone want to take medicine that brought that to a halt?

Dr. Jameson described behaving in ways that reflected John's behavior; erratic, deep mood swings from manic to depressive, argumentative, grandiose, self centered and irresponsible. She described refusing to take her medicine and having constant thoughts of suicide as a way to release the blackness of the bipolar depressive loop. I related to all of it, and began to understand more and more why John behaved as he did when not taking his meds. Reading her book helped me understand that my reactions to John's behavior were normal and that, unless he took his meds and was willing to accept psychiatric counseling, there was very little I could do to really help him. As difficult as that was to know, it was also a relief to understand that my actions—or lack of them--were not the issue. If only I'd known that when I visited the psychiatrist in late 1990.

After my session with the psychiatrist, and for the next three weeks of John's hospitalization, I had time to really ponder what the doctor had told me. So about a month from the initial commitment the day came when John was released from the hospital, and I was there to pick him up and drive him home. He was withdrawn and silent during the ride. I'd no idea what to expect and in fact I was silently terrified about how I would be able to handle him.

With John home, Mary came by the house every couple of days to bring his mail and discuss bank business. In the early days she'd also bring him things to sign. On those days he worked so hard to be like his old self that it wrenched your heart. Her visits were high points for him, but for the rest of the day he'd sleep the sleep of someone totally exhausted. During John's hospitalization, I'd come to the conclusion that barring a miracle he would never be able to resume his role as bank president. Now I began to think about helping him accept the reality that he needed to control his exit by resigning. Convincing him would be a hard sell, but it needed to be done.

Within a few days of his release from the hospital it became apparent to others as well that a decision was going to have to be made about his future. Up to this point the bank directors had been completely supportive. Two directors, Don and Mike, came to visit several times and many of the others phoned every now and then to check on John. Everyone was particularly caring and concerned toward me. But I knew it was over.

Every time I talked to John about resigning his position before the directors were forced to release him he'd become greatly agitated, so I suggested he call our old and dear friend Paul and talk to him about the situation. Paul lived in a nearby town and had worked with John on bank promotions from time to time in both Jackson and Houston. They were great friends and John respected his intellect.

Paul and John went back to the days when John was a banker in Houston. Paul frequently worked on political campaigns as well and was known all over Texas as a gifted campaign strategist. There were many evenings both in Houston and Jackson when Paul, John and I would sit around our kitchen table and argue politics and religion until we were blue in the face. It was great fun. Paul actually helped John and I design our home since he also had the skills of a draftsman.

Paul did come to the house at John's invitation and between the two of us we convinced him to write his resignation. We helped him with the letter and I mailed it the next day. The letter was dated December 13, 1990, a defining moment for John, whose self-esteem and personal identity were aligned with his position as a bank president. In his eyes, if he wasn't bank president then he was nobody. And, although the doctors, his friends and I tried to show him that he was more than what he did, we failed completely.

John was in a great depression at this time, taking several medications—lithium for his bipolar condition, Depakote for paranoia and Prozac for anxiety and depression. The medical establishment believed this particular cocktail was helpful in controlling the major aspects of the traumatic brain injury as well as the bipolar disorder and paranoia. Further research has been done since then, and it's now believed by some that such a combination of meds actually exacerbates all of those conditions.

It was a daily struggle for me to make sure John took his meds as he hated them with a passion. "They make me feel lethargic and dull," he told me. His manic episodes were so euphoric that when the meds kicked in to balance him out it was a huge contrast. We were both concerned that the meds caused his hands to shake so much that it was difficult for him to hold a cup of coffee without spills. He was embarrassed and would often pour his coffee out rather than keep spilling it.

Christmas that year was very grim. That was true of most Christmas seasons during the eight years I remained married to John after the accident. Gary, John and I tried to make the best of it but we couldn't help remembering earlier times when Christmas meant skiing trips to Crested Butte, Beaver Creek and Breckenridge with friends. We remembered the exhilaration of being outdoors, flying down the slopes, and falling into a snow bank. (Or, in my case, nearly making an unintended visit to the kids ski school on the bunny slopes when learning to ski and not knowing how to stop!) There were fond memories of sitting by the fireplace, worn out yet happy at the end of a day on the slopes. But those days were gone. Now we were dealing with a very depressed person who was fast becoming someone we didn't know and didn't like all that much either. That's what transformed the Christmas season into our least favorite time of year, and why Gary and I now plan a Christmas trip almost every year to some place fun to get away from our old memories and the sadness they still bring.

Gary had a hard time getting home for Christmas from Durango, Colorado the first year after John's accident. In fact, we thought he might not make it at all due to the bad weather all over the country that year. Uncharacteristically, we even had ice and snow on the ground in east Texas. Gary was coming by bus because by the time he'd decided to come home it was too late to get an airline reservation. We were there to meet him at the bus station in a nearby town because the bus couldn't get to Jackson. John drove and I remember the roads were so very treacherous. It took us a long time to get to the bus station. I was so glad to see Gary but soon saw to my disappointment that he was more withdrawn than ever. He spent most of the holidays at his friends' homes. I understood--he was still very young, and devastated by his dad's illness. He'd also learned painfully that people seemed to treat him differently once they knew his dad was mentally ill. I experienced some of that as well but not to the degree that Gary did. His way of coping was just to remove himself from the situation at home. It was such a difficult time for both John and me that truthfully I wished I could remove myself as well. When it was time for him to leave, I took Gary back to the bus station in Jackson. John had declined to ride with us because he was so depressed and I believe he just couldn't deal with Gary leaving home once again. As the bus pulled away, I waved goodbye to Gary feeling desolate and very alone.

As 1990 drew to a close I was exhausted, worried and in real emotional pain. Financially, we were in good shape. John had sold our bank stock, which was snapped up quickly by the bank directors. We got top dollar for it and it was wisely invested, so I was grateful for that. On the other hand, John was withdrawing even further into his deep depression, talking very little and moving into a suicidal state of mind. I had a sinking feeling that though 1990 had presented us with many horrors the worst was yet to come.

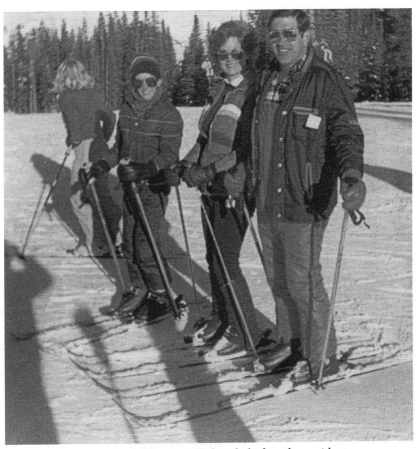

Memories of ski trips to Colorado before the accident.
Crested Butte, CO

13

The Unbelievable and the Unthinkable

Once John resigned, we began what I think of as phase two of his illness. He was drowning in his depression and I knew, even though he denied it, that he wasn't taking the full dosage of his meds. "I hate the way they make me feel," he told me over and over again. I came to the conclusion that if I didn't get him to rally soon he would most certainly kill himself. He'd already threatened to. I was driving to my work in a neighboring city and back every day and worried that I was so far away as he was by himself at home. I'd call him frequently during the day. As I drove into the driveway every evening I wondered who John would be this time—the manic John, or the depressed John? Would I find him lying in a pool of blood, dead from the bullet he kept threatening to put in his head? I'd pray for strength and then drag myself out of the car and into the house to face whatever awaited me.

On one occasion he called me at my office and told me he was just through with everything. He was going to get his gun and put himself out of his horrific misery. "I love you and Gary more than I can say," he told me in a hoarse whisper. "I am so very sorry to bring this on you both." With my heart in my mouth, I talked him down.

"Promise me you won't do anything before I get home," I begged. When he agreed, I ran to my car and drove like a crazy woman.

As I ran through the door, there he was—sitting with the gun in his lap. A strange calm came over me, and I sat and talked with him for a long time and then asked him to put the gun down. I told him how greatly he was loved by both Gary and me. "You'll leave an enormous hole in our lives if you do this," I told him softly. He sobbed and sobbed, telling me over and over he was no good anymore. "John, that's just not true," I replied, listing all the ways he'd been a good husband and father. Finally, he put the gun on the coffee table. Without hesitating, I picked it up and locked it back in the gun cabinet, all the while thanking God he hadn't used it.

That was the first of many times I talked him out of shooting himself. (The obvious solution would have been to remove the guns from the house immediately. I don't know why it took me so long. Although, when I eventually did, it made John furious.)

One evening not long after, he said he had to go down to the corner store to get cigarettes. "Be careful driving," I told him, and thought no more about it. After the suicidal incident with the gun I had talked to the doctor, voicing my suspicions that John wasn't taking his meds, no matter what I tried. "I know he lies to me about taking them," I said. The doctor talked to him, and it seemed to do the trick, even though John was very upset that I'd made the call. However, he did return to his meds, although very soon he was mellowed out to the point that I was worried something wasn't right with the dosage.

When he returned from the store that evening he said very little, sitting almost in a stupor watching TV. About an hour later, as I let our Doberman, Lady, in for the night I realized I hadn't seen our exuberant Doberman puppy, Angel. She was a pure delight. She loved everyone and was an "attack licker." John simply adored her.

I asked him if he knew why she wasn't with Lady. His calm reply was chilling. "Yes, I ran over her on the driveway." Stunned, I yelled, "Oh my God, are you kidding me? Why didn't you tell me immediately when you got back? Did you kill her?" He simply shrugged. "I don't know," he said, turning back to the TV. I raced outside and up the driveway. She'd dragged herself onto the side of the driveway, into the grass. There is no way to describe what I was feeling as I knelt down beside her. Angel turned her beautiful brown eyes to my face and whimpered. Until then I thought my heart had been broken as far as it could go. I was wrong because seeing that precious little dog finished it off.

Still sobbing, I ran back into the house to call our vet, who was a bank customer and a friend. Without hesitation he said he was on his way. I stayed with Angel until he arrived. "I think I can save her, but I need to take her back to my office," he told me. I followed in my car, still trembling. He'd called his assistant, who met us there. Together they worked on Angel while I waited anxiously in the waiting room, crying softly and praying that this sweet baby would be okay.

Finally the vet came out to tell me she would recover but he'd stay with her that night and in all likelihood she would need to stay with him for the next couple of days. I was so grateful but still shaking. I stepped in to see Angel before I left to kiss her nose, look in her eyes and promise her I'd be back. Injured as she was, she licked me—her trademark.

When I got home I found John still watching TV in a stupor. I knelt in front of him. "How in God's name could you run over Angel, and then just leave her to die," I demanded. He looked at me blankly, dragging his gaze from the TV only long enough to tell me he didn't run over her. Still reeling, I called John's doctor. A blood test during our visit to his office the next day confirmed it: John's meds were off, and the doctor quickly adjusted his dosage.

Even when I picked Angel up from the vet clinic and brought her home, John acted as if nothing had really happened. Angel loved him and immediately went to him when she got home. "I love you, Angel," he said as he scratched her head. I added this to my fast-growing list of hair-raising experiences that we'd somehow lived though since his accident. I naively thought the list couldn't be topped.

Barely two weeks later, John ran over Angel again. She'd been healing very nicely when he hit her right hind leg. I went through the same scenario of realizing she was missing, questioning him and him telling me she was hit outside in the driveway. Again I called the vet, who was incredulous. After a two-day stay, I once again brought her home from the clinic, but she was very weak.

One evening not long afterward I went to check on her and bring both dogs in for the night. I quickly realized she was not with Lady and was again missing. This time, John said he'd no idea where she was. I took the flashlight and did a perimeter search but didn't find her. John stayed inside watching his beloved television, refusing to help outside—something he would never have done prior to his accident. I did not sleep at all that night imagining all kinds of gruesome scenarios involving Angel. John was awake much of the night too—but most nights didn't go to bed until very late anyway, and sometimes he didn't sleep for days (which I later learned is a marker for bipolar disorder.) He definitely didn't seem at all concerned that Angel was missing. However, the next day he did agree to help search for her. It was a cloudy gray day, which entirely matched our mood. We saddled our horses and rode the entire 55 acres but found no sign of her. In fact, we never found her, and I became convinced that in her weakened condition the coyotes who frequented our property (which is why we brought the dogs in at night) had found her in such a weakened condition she couldn't defend herself and they simply dragged her off, killed and ate her.

When a couple of days had elapsed with no Angel, I came home one day after work and found John with his head in his hands crying. When I asked him what was wrong he looked at me with such misery. "Angel's gone and she's not coming back." He still had no conscious understanding of his role in her disappearance. My own feelings were raw so we sat and cried together, only I wasn't just crying for Angel. My tears were for my husband as well. The guilt I felt for ever letting Angel out of the house after he hit her the second time was enormous. *If only I'd left her on her bed inside. If only I'd been more vigilant.* So the accusatory voice of guilt went on inside my head. It would be a very long time before I could let myself off of the hook for her death. After that single afternoon of grieving together for our puppy, John never mentioned her again.

14
Getting John Professionally Engaged

In the early spring of 1991 I had an inspired idea about how I might get John redirected. His depression was palpable and I felt an urgency to find a way to bring him out of it because he still talked of killing himself and as we went along I felt he might be getting closer to making good on his threats. He loved technology (although, compared with today, it was still relatively primitive) and there was a spare Classic Apple computer in my office so I took it home to him. "I'll show you what little I know about it, then it's up to you," I said. As I handed him the manual he lit up like a Christmas tree. "Take the next couple of days to play around with it," I said. "If you like it, we can buy our own." He fell in love immediately, so we bought one. Thankfully, it had the desired effect and before long he told me he'd like to start his own consulting business.

His idea seemed the answer to my prayers. I'd been searching for a way to get him to see himself as something other than a banker so he could explore where else he could use his skills and intellect. His mental state was such that while he wasn't as quick as he used to be, he still retained his ability to think at a high level if given more time. His business idea was to provide banks with customized products and services manuals, as he felt there was no one filling that niche.

I encouraged him to develop his idea. He began with the products and services manual he'd created while bank president, throwing himself into creating a prototype, doing all of the work to get the manual from hard copy into the computer. At night I'd help him proofread and edit.

John had always been a perfectionist and was more so now but at last his days were filled with what he recognized as productive, creative work. He was excited about life again, and the ideas kept on coming. "You know, this won't be of any value unless I also develop a training component to teach bankers how to use their manual," he told me after he'd finished the prototype. "Now, I'm not a teacher but you are. You've had lots of experience training and teaching adults as well as kids. Do you think you can design a training linked to the customized manual?" I didn't hesitate. "Of course," I said. It was an easy decision, because I love doing that kind of thing. In truth, I also loved the idea of him being excited about a project, and getting to work on it with him. So we began.

After I got home each evening I worked on the training design. When I showed him what I'd done, he was thrilled. And then he told me his new idea. "You know I can't deliver this training—but you can. What do you think? I'll be there as your subject matter expert who explains the technical parts of banking you don't know." Now it was my turn to be thrilled. As calmly as I could, I said I was up for the challenge.

He contacted Paul and together we three designed a brochure for the new business. Nicholson and Associates was officially incorporated in the fall of 1991. John then began to contact banker friends across the country. The first person to sign up was his friend Steve in Alabama who had been on the horse packing trips and witnessed the accident. We set the training for a Saturday and it was a whopping success.

I loved doing the training, and the positive response from the participants was overwhelming. They told me they'd never had so much fun learning nor had it ever been so easy. I used many teaching strategies they'd never experienced, designed to lock in initial learning and transfer it to long-term memory. I was always both amused and sad that when we trained leaders of million (and sometimes even billion) dollar institutions that they'd arrive at the training location looking like fearful eight-year-olds on the first day of school, not knowing what to expect. Unfortunately, that fear harkened back to their school days, when some members of my profession had done their best to make learning painful. I knew our training would be a learning experience for them like no other because, besides getting John productive again It was also the perfect opportunity for me to undo some of the learning damage I'd frequently seen when teaching adults.

Steve told his banker friends how successful we'd been at his bank. Word soon spread and for about the next year John got steady orders from bankers across the country to create customized manuals. We'd travel on Friday night after I got off work at the school district, do Saturday trainings, then travel home Saturday night or Sunday. Monday morning I'd go back to work. It was exhilarating but also exhausting. We had great fun traveling to our training locations, staying at nice hotels, eating in great restaurants, and enjoying each other's company. It was almost like it used to be. However, I soon began to see that John was unhappy and cracks began to show. He was going downhill again.

There were many reasons for his downward spiral. It was a combination of him not taking his meds consistently, taking less than prescribed, refusing much needed psychiatric counseling, and his emerging resentment of me. He knew it was ridiculous to resent the fact that, unlike him, I was so at home in front of an audience and loved teaching. But he couldn't help himself. I realized the minute the resentment set in, and immediately sat him down to talk to me about it.

He denied how he was feeling at first, and I didn't push. But then his feelings began to impact the trainings. The evaluations of my work were still very good but gradually people began to notice, and comment on, John's growing lack of interest. I knew I had to try to continue to keep him involved while responding to the changes our participants were requesting. He'd read the evaluations and see the difference between his and mine. I was distraught that these were so devastating to him. I talked to him about not even doing evaluations. However, he rejected that unequivocally. So I determined I couldn't tell him that things were just great when they needed to be adjusted. I reasoned that to do so would be to dishonor him and certainly cause him to lose clients.

Finally, the right time came and for whatever reason he was open to a discussion. He told me one of the things he'd always loved about me was the way I handle people. "You're a natural at public speaking and teaching, Donna and I love you for it," he said with tears in his eyes. "The problem is, I'm no longer who I was." That was to be the closest he ever came to admitting he was mentally ill.

I went to bed that night with a very heavy heart wondering what I could do to make things better for John. Suddenly I had one of those "aha!" moments, which remains with me today. In that moment I realized you should never be less of who you are so someone else can be more of who they want to be. Nor could you be. Clarity vanished as fast as it had arrived. "How can you be so selfish?" my inner voice demanded. Confused, I began second guessing myself. *Surely I can tone things down so the man I love won't feel so threatened or suffer more than he is already.*

I chewed on that for several days and in the end I knew I was right the first time: you cannot be less of who you are so someone else can be more of who they want to be. That would most certainly be dishonoring of both John and me. One evening I brought the subject up again, only this time I had some ideas about what would make John comfortable in his role while still adding value to the business. I never got to share those ideas because he told me in a threatening voice I'd never heard from him before that he "damn well wasn't interested." That's when I began to notice his personality was shifting toward something much darker. Day by day he became more fractious, demanding and short tempered.

He continued to pass his latest manual to me to proofread. I'd make corrections and take it back to him. He'd start to work on the changes, and then just explode in fury. He'd charge through the house, find me and start complaining that he couldn't read my writing. "By God, if you're going to do my proofreading you'd better learn to write better!" My initial response was to get calmer as he got more agitated. Lowering my voice, I'd point out that my handwriting was clear and hadn't changed from the day I began doing his proofreading and editing. (This of course was long before the word processing capabilities we have today, spell and grammar check and the wonderful cut and paste feature.)

I held my own resentment at bay for a very long time trying to learn to deal with this new twist in his illness in a productive way. However, here I was commuting 45 minutes each way to work every day, handling the immense pressure of my professional responsibilities, coming home, cooking dinner, cleaning up and then working on his business with him until late at night. Then getting up the next morning and doing it all over.

One evening when he started in with the same obnoxious behavior I'd reached the end of my rope and let him have it with both barrels. I'm naturally articulate, but when I'm riled, I'm articulate in the extreme. I imagine if I'd been on the outside looking into our arguments I would have cringed at my scathing response to John.

This continued for many weeks and months and I was so miserable, while he was sinking further and further into depression. He was increasingly aloof and I spent the rest of the year trying to figure out how to get him back to some balance. We were still doing seminars but I was now carrying most of the load as John shrank more and more from the public part of our work. He was still involved in writing the manuals but had lost all interest in, and even dreaded, the seminars. I asked him if he wanted to do away with them. He seemed surprised, saying, "No, that's the best part of the business and it's probably why we keep getting new clients."

Shortly after this conversation, John decided that having an exhibit booth at professional conferences would help the business. He created the marketing materials and, all credit to him, they were first class. He would drive or fly to wherever the latest exhibit venue was located. I stayed on pins and needles with worry for him in this latest venture. It was painfully evident this wasn't something John really liked to do or was comfortable with.

As 1991 came to a close, I felt he was in such a deep dark hole that it was now impossible for me to reach him.

15
Off to Colorado

I had dared to dream that 1992 would bring us some hope and certainly a brighter future but I also had deep doubts that would be the case. In fact, as it turned out, 1992 was one of the most frustrating and hopeless times in both our lives. It was a year of maddening repetition of the gigantic highs and lows associated with his bipolar, of my not knowing which way to jump, and coming to the frustrating conclusion that I couldn't help John because he steadfastly refused to avail himself of psychiatric help. Ironically, even though I knew all of this, I could not seem to let go of the desperate desire and personal need to help him—if I could only figure out how. It was so obvious that he needed to work with a psychologist or a psychiatrist as he was drowning in depression and hopelessness.

I continued to try and persuade him. I once again begged him to call Dr. McNamara, or let me on his behalf. John had begrudgingly trusted the doctor but he knew he was not going to be able to push him around nor bamboozle him with his charm. In fact, Dr. McNamara told me while John was in the hospital that John used this strategy frequently when things got too intense. But, as Dr. McNamara told me, "I just made him face it." That may explain why John didn't want to deal with him after he came home. However, anything other than a strong figure would not have worked with him. John would simply have overpowered any other doctor with his intellect and his strong will, which would not have been helpful at all because he needed to face the issues to heal.

I knew we were getting much closer to John carrying out his threat to commit suicide. In fact, he had at least two incidents that year where I stopped him from killing himself. Both times he had his gun cocked and ready when I found him, once in the garage and once in the barn. Each time I talked him out of it by pointing out how much he was needed as a father to Gary and a husband to me. And each time he reluctantly gave me the gun, telling me again through tears he was an awful father and husband.

He also continued cycling between taking his meds, taking only partial dosages and not taking them at all. There were times when I was so frustrated and discouraged that I screamed at God for putting us in this position because I was still holding Him accountable. I certainly was no closer to "why" than I had been when the accident occurred. Nothing seemed to work and I felt we were stuck in this never-ending cycle. I was working hard not to lose my own sanity and to continue to provide John the stability I still felt he needed.

As the year came to a close and we were moving into 1993 I was glad to see it arrive, and again dared to hope it would provide something different. Having hope, as tremulous as it was, provided one of the few things that I had control over back then, and I hung to it for dear life, despite the many setbacks, steadfastly denying the proof before my own eyes as to just how hopeless things were. Irrational? Yes. But it got me through.

In fact, 1993 did bring with it a glimmer of hope, as I was offered a deputy superintendent position for an upscale district in the Dallas metro area through a friend who was the superintendent there. I didn't immediately tell John because I wanted to talk to Dr. McNamara first. I told the doctor that the offer would require us to relocate, and that I thought this might be good for John. Frankly, I was desperate for solutions and felt time was of the essence. However,

Dr. McNamara cautioned against moving John this soon after the accident. He said there would come a time when it would be very therapeutic for him but didn't think we were there yet.

I was crushed but I trusted Dr. McNamara, so I told my friend I couldn't accept. Still, her offer got me thinking, and I began talking to John about the possibility of getting out of Jackson at some point. At first he backed up from it, concerned about what he would do in a strange place. I didn't push but quietly started looking in my professional job listings to see what might be a fit for us. Then one day John totally surprised me by suggesting that I start looking for superintendent positions out of state, and just retire from Texas. Ever my mentor and supporter he told me there was just not anything like being the boss. We both knew that I had the credentials to be a superintendent, but as I'd told him before, I didn't want to go in that direction. Being superintendent is about school boards, budgets, bond issues and all the stuff that takes you away from kids. "And I'm all about the kids," I reminded John.

He took my pushback in stride. "Donna, you have so much obvious administrative talent you need to be the boss," he told me. "You can be a superintendent and still make it about kids."

Of course, he wanted me to look in Colorado so we could live in his favorite state. I balked for a while and then half-heartedly applied to some districts in Colorado Springs because that's where he really wanted to live. All three districts I applied to interviewed me, and I ended up in their final round. However, after interviewing with the board and staff of all three, I just knew I didn't want to work there so removed my name from consideration.

John respected my decisions and kept encouraging me to keep interviewing. I continued interviewing in places he thought he'd like to live, like Montana, Wyoming and Utah, yet always removed my name after interviewing and knowing it wasn't a fit for me. He didn't get discouraged and in fact began to come out of his depression. In the beginning this was encouraging. Once I accepted the invitation to interview, he'd set about researching the area, the district, and all of the pertinent information he could gather providing me with what I needed when I interviewed. We were once again partners and his self-esteem seemed to be coming back. I was thrilled and encouraged him to keep helping me.

For the next several months, John kept on searching for jobs for me, escalating the pressure to accept a position. I tried to be patient and share my career but I was fast getting more and more uncomfortable with his intensity. He was clearly moving across the line between just helping me to identifying completely, as if it were his own career search. I knew that wasn't healthy for him, and I worried that when I had to put my foot down with him he'd come unglued again. I felt I was walking on egg shells. And, while my heart hurt for him, I also began to feel real resentment.

Finally, that summer I saw a position opening in Beaverton, Ore. where a friend of mine was the superintendent. I called her and she was delighted to know of my interest and had me fly out immediately to talk to her and the staff about her deputy superintendent position. During my visit I learned that a large part of the job involved interfacing with the district's powerful union. While I knew I could have done that effectively I also knew I didn't want to spend my time doing it.

When John heard I'd turned the job down, he didn't get discouraged and just kept on "managing" potential places for me to interview. This was his new job and he took it very seriously. I was more uncomfortable by the day with the extreme control he was trying to exert on my career, so I began to be less accommodating to his suggestions. When he presented me with a list of places I refused to apply unless they really appealed to me. That didn't go down well, and for the first time he snapped at me. "You can't carry on being so picky, and keep walking away from all of these places where they want you but you don't want them," he said with a glare. "I can keep walking away until doomsday if I feel it's not the right place for me to work," I flashed back. "May I remind you, I have a job, no one is pushing me out and I will jolly well retire and move on when I decide the time is right!" After that spat, John became very quiet and withdrawn for a few days, which filled me with guilt but I absolutely knew I'd done the right thing. That kept me moving forward.

In October, the Assistant Superintendent for Human Resources of Academy District 20 in Colorado Springs called. I was at work so John answered. She told him they had an opening for a deputy superintendent and wanted to talk to me about it. By the time I got home John was very excited. She'd left her home number so I called that evening, and we hit it off immediately. It was as if we'd known each other forever. "Would you be interested in anything other than the superintendency?" she asked. "Funny that you ask that question," I replied. "Truth be told, my goal really isn't to be a superintendent, so I'm greatly interested."

I flew up twice for interviews, hit a home run with all of the interviewing groups and was offered the job. When I accepted John was beside himself with joy. Yet, despite all the excitement, the nature of his joy concerned me because he talked and acted as if he'd just accepted a new job instead of me. His continuing ownership and possessiveness of my job was a growing issue between us and he was often sullen and withdrawn when I confronted him about it.

It was difficult to understand why John would want to move to Colorado, the place where his life-altering accident had occurred. Yet he did, and so began what I think of as phase three of our post-accident lives; phase one being the accident and all of the surrounding drama; phase two being John's resignation from the bank and building his consulting business and now the beginning of phase three: our move to Colorado.

16
The Move From Hell

My new job started the first week of January 1994 so for the remainder of 1993 we began the uprooting process. I was still working, so John and Gary—who was a tremendous help—began organizing the many moving parts of our departure. Gary was again living at home but he planned to enlist in the military after he got us to Colorado, although he wasn't sure which branch.

Our move began with selling the cows and paring down our horses to three. It was a bittersweet time for John because, even though he was completely committed to the move, when we loaded the cows to take them to the sale barn he was very emotional. Selling off our horses was just as emotional for him. We'd decided to lease our home and property in the short term until we could get it sold and to leave our three remaining horses, Skip, Red and Dynamite with the Jackson Sheriff who volunteered to pasture them with his horses until we came back in April to get them. John had found a house to lease in Colorado Springs with about three acres and a barn but it needed some work well before we would be ready to bring the horses up.

Early one morning in December 1993 we drove out of our driveway with John in his truck pulling the horse trailer, Gary driving his little gray truck pulling a flat bed trailer and me in the car. Our Doberman, Lady, and our old cat, Rags, were with John. I had our young cat GC with me and he rode in my lap all the way. I couldn't help thinking back to almost three years ago when another convoy of trucks had driven down the same driveway early in the morning with three men and horses also headed for Colorado. An adventure that precipitated this one.

Our trip to Colorado was a complete nightmare, with John nervous, jumpy and manic. He was more irritable than he'd ever been, and was on Gary's case and mine from the time he got up until the time he went to bed. We could do nothing right. He was short- tempered, stressed and totally unaware that he was making our lives very difficult. I was constantly trying to make peace between Gary and John, while hanging on to what patience I had left. Nothing Gary did was right in John's mind and everything that went wrong could be attributed to Gary. In fact, Gary was remarkably patient with his dad given the circumstances. I found myself losing my temper more and more, and lashing back at John. When I did, he'd take his anger and rage inside, refusing to talk. I just kept comforting myself that this would all be over soon. Moving is a big stressor under normal circumstances. It's off the charts with someone who is mentally ill.

We finally arrived in Colorado Springs and things began to get better as we gradually settled in to our new house. I was immensely busy learning my new job and worked long hours, leaving Gary and John free to repair their relationship. Shortly after our move John bought a Suzuki and together they explored the mountains. Gary recalls those as some of the best times they ever had together.

Looking back, it was always one step forward, two steps back with John's moods in those days. However, he did help Gary select the Navy as the branch of the service that offered him the best opportunities. Now, bit by bit, he began to withdraw as the day for Gary's departure for boot camp came. (He was headed to Orlando, Fla. for basic training.) I was sad as well but I knew our son needed to find his way, and this was just another step toward his growing up. Grief had already begun to settle in with John and the day he took Gary to the airport was a sad one for him indeed. When I came home from work I found him in a darkened room, distraught. Dr. McNamara had told me that when a bipolar disordered person has their routine disturbed the result can be exactly what I was seeing from John. He also told me that loss of any kind would send him into a tailspin, and it could either be manic or depressive.

When I was finally able to get John to talk to me he said he had so many regrets about not being as good a father as he should have been to Gary. However, he never mentioned how horribly he had treated Gary on the trip to Colorado. When I mentioned it, he gave me a blank look. It validated once more what I had already observed—when he was in a manic frenzy he seldom remembered much.

After being so deeply depressed for a couple of weeks John started to emerge and I began to see the now recognizable pattern of slow ascension to manic behavior. I asked him if he was taking his medicine and he barked back at me that he certainly was. I soon discovered that he was only taking half his dosage, so I confronted him and he started taking the full amount. That began a time of relative calm, which was a welcome relief after so many years of turmoil.

During our peaceful period we began the search for land in the area so we could build a new home and replicate the ranch life we'd had in Texas. It was such fun and we ended up with 140 acres in the shadow of Pikes Peak, with rolling hills and breath-taking views of the Peak and the Front Range.

Once John got busy building a barn, repairing fences and drawing plans for our new home he ceased to be so possessive about my career and we rocked along very happily. He purchased a tractor and many summer evenings, when the sky was so beautiful it took your breath away and the air had such a lovely crisp breeze to it, I'd ride on the back of the tractor with him, just as I had in Texas. We were very close at those times and it almost seemed like our lives might begin to resemble the one we'd had before the accident.

We laughed and just enjoyed being together. I remember feeling hugely grateful for my blessings at these times and thanking God for watching over us and bringing us safely to this point.

Many weekends we'd trailer the horses to the mountains and ride to our hearts' content. It was amazing to me that John would ever want to ride again, yet it was as if he'd never had the accident. He continued to love horses and want to ride and enjoy them. I was nervous at first as he began to ride again for fear something else would happen to him but he was relaxed. As a young boy growing up in Houston he'd saved his money for a horse. His family lived very near Rice University so there would be no buying a horse to keep at home. But that didn't stop him from solving the problem. He found stables located where today's Astrodome stands and arranged to board his horse on what was still pastureland when he was growing up. He would ride his bike to the stables every day after school. The horse was black and he named him Dynamite. John simply had a deeply engrained, life-long love of horses that wasn't shaken by his accident.

On one of our horse-riding trips to the mountains near Colorado Springs we climbed to 11,000 feet and camped just under the summit right near a rushing creek. We hobbled the horses at night near our cots and it was wonderful. We had long, deep talks and planned our new home. It was an exciting time and I desperately hoped that we had passed through the worst.

Then I began to once again see the signs that John wasn't taking his medicine. Once again I confronted him. Once again he denied it and lashed out at me verbally. I held my ground and he promised to get back on the meds.

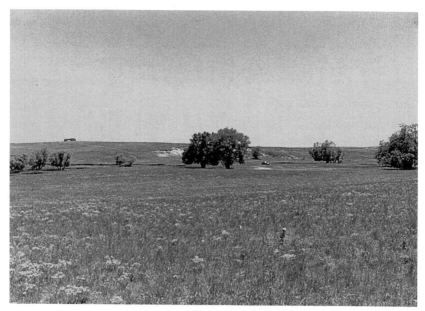

The Colorado ranch.

17
It Just Keeps Getting Worse

One day not long after our horse-riding trip to the mountains we learned that the people we'd leased our Colorado home from had decided to renovate it in preparation for putting it on the market. We knew two things—we didn't want to buy the home and we most certainly did not want to live in it while it was being renovated.

So we scouted around for another house to lease until our own new home was finished, although it wasn't easy as there weren't a lot of lease houses available that we liked. As we began to plan another move less than a year after moving from Texas, John's anxiety level escalated. Finding a house took a while, and by the time we finally got to moving day and began loading the U-Haul he was once again frantic, jumpy and manic. We had some high school boys from my school district helping us and he was every bit as pushy and overbearing toward them as he had been to our son during our initial move to Colorado. I remember taking him aside and reading him the riot act for his behavior. After that he apologized to the boys and held himself at bay for the rest of the move, but just barely.

Shortly after that second move I saw him skyrocket to a manic state and I knew we were in for another full-blown manic episode, I just didn't know what form it was about to take. I vividly remember one incident that just about did me in. I knew John was looking for help clearing the land we'd bought so we could start construction on our new house. As I soon learned, he went looking for that help at the Star of Hope Mission in downtown Colorado Springs. I came home one evening from work to find a complete stranger standing in my living room—alone, as John had gone out to his truck. I could smell him the minute I got in the house. It was a mix of the rankest body odor and cheap alcohol.

He looked as if he'd not slept in days, had a menacing scowl on his face, and I wouldn't have been surprised to see him raise a gun at me, that's how scary he looked. He was about to take a bath, and John had invited him to spend the night in our guest bedroom. John appeared just before I totally lost it, and I asked him to go back outside so we could speak privately. "What were you thinking, bringing this man into our home?" I asked. "Do you know him?" He'd picked him up about an hour earlier at the Mission, John told me calmly. "He smelled bad, so I thought he needed a bath and some sleep before we got started," John explained casually. "He's been on a drinking binge for the last few days."

"What do you know about his background and situation?" I asked. Hearing that the folks at the Mission had told John the man had a criminal record really sent me around the bend. I took a deep breath. "This is not going to happen," I said, as patiently as I could—the frustration bubbling inside. Taking a bath in our home was one thing I explained, but given his criminal record, spending the night in our home while we slept was worse than bad judgment. Prior to his accident, John might have helped the man but would never have brought him to our home. I tried to get him to see that, at best, the man could steal from us and, at worst, kill us while we slept in our bed. John slowly began to see my point, and loaded the man up to return him to the Mission.

While he was gone, I tried to look at what had just happened in as rational a manner as I could, and to see it through John's eyes and heart. I knew that all of our married life he had been sensitive to and respectful of others in need. He'd reached out to many people along the way to offer his help. As a matter of fact, this was one of the personal qualities that made me love him. However, I had seen this quality as well as his normally excellent judgment and decision-making obliterated by his illness. Somewhere inside the stranger he had become he was still a person of deep compassion. It was almost unbearable to realize that, though he put the two of us at risk by inviting this man into our home, his intentions were pure. Once again I'd had to be the "bad guy," and once again I added that to my burden of guilt.

A few days after my encounter with the scary stranger, I realized that John had spent $12,000 in 48 hours before I discovered it and stopped him. I'd left my office one day to join John at our new home site. As I drove up, all I could see were stacks and stacks of building materials. Our new home was to be a small one, and unless he'd decided to build a mansion, there was no way we would ever need what I now saw. "Why did you buy so much?" I asked. "Simple," came the reply. "You never know what you might need. And anyway, I'm sure I will need it all." I asked to see the receipts for everything, and John reluctantly handed them to me as we walked off to inspect his inventory. As I calculated the total it took my breath away.

Since his accident I'd observed that John the conservative banker was never really lost, even though most bipolar disordered people while in a manic episode give money away because it feels like they have an inexhaustible supply of it. Not John. Somehow he had retained his fiscal responsibility because it was so deeply ingrained. Until this incident. He and I had a huge argument, with me warning him I knew he'd again stopped taking his meds. "From now on you had better take them," I yelled. I considered talking to his doctor and starting the process of commitment for the second time but decided John hadn't gotten to that level of behavior; he was just on the edge of it. Or so I thought.

Unfortunately, not long after that, he did go over the edge, continuing to hire all kinds of help, and buying more building materials.

All told, he had bought about $20, 000 dollars worth, most of which I was thankfully able to get returned. In his right mind he would never have spent money so recklessly.

I was just exhausted with worry about him and with not knowing if I should commit him again or not. It might sound like an obvious decision to make given this incident, but when you have to commit someone to a mental hospital it does something to you and you will do almost anything to avoid repeating it. However, I finally decided that I would try one more time to get his attention in a way he would not miss. If that failed, I told myself, then I'd have no choice. He recognized that I was angrier this time with him than I had ever been. I was beyond furious, and laid the law down as never before, telling him I wouldn't tolerate his lack of responsibility when it came to taking his medicine. "I won't even blink an eyelash about committing you to a mental hospital again if you don't get back on those meds and stay on them," I told him in no uncertain terms. This time he was surly and angry. "You can't tell me what to do. Not about anything," he raged. However, as he stalked away I knew he would heed my warning. His hatred and fear of mental hospitals went back years, to the time he'd committed his own mother.

My harsh words may have successfully made a believer out of John, but they left me feeling vulnerable once more, gripped with guilt at being so stern with him and devastated that again we were at this juncture. I now realized that each manic episode was chipping away at him, filling him each time with more rage and more hate, escalating his personality disorder beyond the point of return.

His paranoia took center stage as it never had before. He was distrustful of me without any reason and often accused me of ridiculous acts. Yes, I continued to confront him, but down deep I was for the first time feeling that I might not be safe with him. Gary came home at Christmas time that year and he saw the same behavior. John was so hateful he made me cry—and that is hard to do. Gary was infuriated, and the two had strong words until John eventually backed down. Seeing this unfold before me, I remembered what the psychiatrist in Texas had said when I'd asked if bipolar people get violent. "Some do, some don't." Given John's current behavior, I knew I had decisions to make.

Even though my personal life was going steadily downhill my professional life was reaching new heights. I loved my new job. The Academy school district in Colorado Springs has three of its 20 campuses on the campus of the United States Air Force Academy. No other public school system in the country has such a unique relationship with a Service Academy. John was immensely proud that I'd been recruited by such an outstanding district, although he often spoke as if he was the one who'd been recruited. I did some of my best professional work there and made some lifelong friends whom I cherish to this day. Yet, as 1994 came to a close, I was growing more and more concerned about my life with John.

Then in February the school district where we lived, just adjacent to the one I worked for, had an opening for a superintendent. It was growing at a rate of 12% a year, needed new schools but hadn't been able to pass a bond issue despite six attempts. It wasn't a rich district and had suffered from a long history of bad boards plus a revolving door of superintendents. I was very happy as the Deputy Superintendent for the Academy District 20 and had no desire to apply for any new position, let alone the superintendent's position in the district where I lived. However, I began to have local parents, teachers and students from the district ask if I would apply because they needed so much help. They told me they had no technology, not enough books and they believed there was something bad going on with the district's money. It all added up to an utter lack of trust in the district administrators and the board.

The more I got lobbied to apply, and the more I checked into the history of the district, the more I resisted the pressure to apply. John, always my mentor and pushing me to stretch my wings in leadership, almost ordered me to apply. Gone was my subtle mentor of the past. We had words more than once, with me warning John to back off and leave me alone to make the decision. Once again he was trying to hijack my career.

My decision to apply was made when students kept telling me they were in crowded schools and they weren't getting a very good education. I have a history of building trust with school communities very quickly, and have used it to move my agenda for kids more than once. And I knew how to use it to get a bond issue passed for new schools. So nothing about this new position seemed insurmountable even though I knew it wouldn't be easy.

John was beyond delighted and began to talk in terms of when *we* get the superintendent's position we can do thus and so. I let it go sometimes but when I corrected him it would set his temper off, then he'd get hurt and pout, which made me feel mean and guilty. Little wonder I'd sometimes let his comments slide.

I interviewed with the board twice and accepted their offer of a three-year contract in late March 1995. I began to plan for my transition out of Academy with lots of tears and well wishes from my school district family. John was on a high just to think that I was going to be the superintendent.

18
The Bottom Falls Out

On July 1, 1995 I began my job as superintendent. I knew the priority was to build trust with my community where none existed, so I divided my district into quadrants and designed my plan like a political campaign. I divided those quadrants into blocks with block captains who would host neighborhood coffees for me. It was John who helped me with this strategy, recalling it from the days when he'd been active in Houston politics as a young man.

The bond election for the school district was set for the same day as the general election, November 7. Between July 1 and November 7, I spent over 300 hours in neighborhood coffees getting to know my community, articulating the vision I had for their kids and the school district that served them. They were stunned that a superintendent and her principals would actually bring the debate to them and sit in their homes and talk to them neighbor—to-neighbor. John wanted to do the coffees with me so much, but I knew that was a bad idea and told him so as kindly and firmly as I could. He wasn't happy with me and began to swing between manic and depressive as I continued to work my community without him.

My guilt was at an all-time high, knowing he felt so adrift and unconnected. Here he was, forever separated from the profession he loved and had been so obviously successful in. Here I was, further separating him from an opportunity to use his enormous skill with people. My compassion for how he was feeling hurt to the bone. Thank goodness my common sense prevailed.

Three weeks into my tenure, which was about the middle of July, my Chief Financial Officer came into my office bringing with her two large file folders. "This is going to stun you," she said by way of kicking off the subject. She'd shown the contents of these same file folders to my two predecessors, who had both stayed about two years, and yet they had both determined not to act on the information. Needless to say, by now she had my full attention. "There is overwhelming evidence that the board is criminally liable for the way they've spent public monies," she continued. "I feel obligated to bring this information to light, and do not want to be seen as complicit."

"Under no circumstance will I look the other way," I told the CFO. "Even though the board will likely end up firing me."

John was simply stricken when I told him what had happened, and what I proposed to do about it. He definitely supported me in doing the right thing, but his heart was just sick. His opinion on how I ought to handle things coincided with my plan, and he rose to the occasion, becoming my greatest support even while fighting the pull of his depression. I recognized then and even more so later how much internal character he had because, as I grew to understand the kind of depression a bipolar person experiences, I could see what fighting to keep from sinking into the depths of depression had to have cost him. He knew he could not support me when he fell off into that black hole so he fought valiantly to get enough traction to prevent it. However, the nature of bipolar depression is beyond description and like a giant magnet there came a point where no matter how hard he struggled to hang on to the edge of darkness, he was sucked into it.

I called the board president in the next day and the CFO supported me as I told him I knew what he and the board had been up to and we began to show him the contents of the file folders. We didn't get very far with that before he ordered me to put the file folders back in the file cabinet and shut my mouth. "And you can do the same," he demanded, turning to the CFO. I told him I would not help him hide the board's wrongdoing and most certainly would not be quiet about what they'd done. "You've got three choices," I told him icily. I would take the evidence to the District Attorney, he could take it, or we would go together.

"You're forgetting the fourth choice," he shot back. "You do as I said in the first place: put the folders away and keep quiet before the board fires you." I calmly replied that was not a choice as far as I was concerned. "You'll just have to do what you feel you have to do. My plan is to take this to the D.A. on November 8th." I'd already decided to wait to turn the board in until the day after the bond election because I didn't want any adverse publicity to get in the way of that election—even though I knew we'd now pass it. He threatened me once again with firing before leaving. "Knock your lights out," were my parting words as he stormed out.

When I went home that evening and told John he poured me a glass of wine and reassured me I'd done the right thing. He was in his element, and seemed almost normal. I was thankful for small mercies.

Things began to unravel quickly. Shortly after the meeting in my office, the board president began a campaign of sexual harassment directed at me, launching it at a dinner hosted by our bond counsel. We'd gathered to discuss the financial and legal obligations of the board and superintendent in a bond issue as well as strategies we would need to consider when it passed. Spouses were invited so John was there. I was seated between the board president and John. When the board president made his move, John had his back to me, talking to the person on his other side. That, thank goodness, meant he was unable to see the board president put his hand on my arm and rub it up and down. "Leave -me -alone," I whispered, enunciating each word through clenched teeth as I quickly pushed him away.

On the way home I debated whether to tell John. He'd become so volatile, and I knew this would really push his buttons. He'd fought so hard to stay out of the depths of depression that he'd begun swinging toward the manic side. He was already showing signs of moving into the manic loop anyway and I knew this would only escalate it. So, I didn't tell him that night.

As the days rolled by, the board president began to accelerate his campaign. I'd hear direct from the parents about the inappropriate remarks he'd make in public about my body. I told them to document what they heard, but it got to the point that I knew I was going to have to do something more. I also knew I needed to tell John because soon I would need to take legal action. The time came one evening when we were having a glass of wine on the back deck and he seemed pretty stable and in a good mood. As I calmly told him what was going on, he erupted. "I'm going to go get my gun and put that little son of a bitch out of his misery!" he yelled. In an instant I regretted telling him. It took a while, but when he'd calmed down I asked him what I should do. "It's simple, Donna," he told me. "You've got to confront him about his behavior, and after the election we have to get an attorney and stop him, even if we have to sue him."

He was right, of course. But in all of my life no one had ever come close to treating me this way and I couldn't stop myself from wondering what I had done to bring this behavior on myself. Intellectually, I knew better but I also didn't know how to deal with my feelings about it appropriately, besides knowing it was wrong. John quickly set me straight about what sexual harassment is all about—power. That evening, despite the topic, was another increasingly rare and precious time together.

Election Day dawned, and I knew without a doubt that our bond issue would pass. My community had banded together on behalf of their kids and helped me plan the Get Out the Vote phase so I knew we would have plenty of yes votes. John and I went to the county office to await the election returns along with the bond issue steering committee. He was in great spirits and though a bit expansive he was within normal bounds with it. About 9:00 pm it was clear we had won! The margin was three to one in an election with 27 taxing initiatives on the ballot, all of which went down in flames except our bond issue. John was elated and we all celebrated. The bond campaign had been grueling and I had finally found an appropriate role for John to play in designing the campaign strategy. He was good at that and he'd worked with Paul, the expert and friend who had helped craft John's resignation from the bank in Jackson. So it was John's victory as well.

However, the good feelings the passage of the bond issue had produced were about to be dashed. The day after the election, as I had promised, I called the board president to remind him of what I was going to do with the incriminating evidence of the board's malfeasance. I once again reviewed his option of turning himself and the board in to the D.A. or going with me to deliver the file folders. He once again threatened to lead the board to fire me if I took the folders out of the central office and once again told me to put them away and shut up. He also got in one last sexually harassing comment, which I documented for use later. Once I hung up I drove to the D.A.'s office and turned the files over.

He was stunned and kept shaking his head in disbelief at the evidence. He finally explained the process, which would take about six months to complete. It included an investigation to substantiate the contents of the files and the CFO's explanation of what she knew first hand. I will always love and respect the CFO because in exposing the board she put her own job at great risk. Yet she was bound and determined to do the right thing. We both knew there would be consequences for our decision to blow the whistle on the board and we knew it would come soon.

At home that night John agreed there was nothing else I could have done. His mood after the exhilaration of the day before was subdued. He was very quiet and though I probed gently as to how he felt he just didn't want to talk, although he agreed that we needed to find an attorney to discuss the sexual harassment issue. His depression was once more taking hold, as now we'd won the election, he felt left out and useless again.

PART FOUR

THIS JUST CAN'T BE HAPPENING

19
Doing the Right Thing is Painful

In early December of 1995, without my knowledge, the school district's board president set up an illegal meeting with the other board members. My own administrative assistant, who was also the board secretary, was helping the board behind my back, something I didn't learn until after the fact. The meeting was illegal for a couple of reasons. In the first place, it wasn't posted within the legal time requirements. The board also went into closed executive session even though their reasons for doing so didn't meet the legal criteria.

Little wonder there was such cloak and dagger shenanigans, as it turned out what they were hatching behind those closed doors was their plan to fire me. Now, while it is one thing to hatch a plan in an executive session, it is completely illegal to take any kind of action during that executive session. Actions must be taken in an open legally posted session. Despite that, the board began by changing the superintendent's evaluation format so it would be easier to get rid of me. They then proceeded to use the new format to evaluate my performance. Once that was done, they voted to terminate my contract. All behind those closed doors.

It wasn't by any means the first time they'd violated the laws governing public officials and meeting protocols. Throughout the fall of 1995 they'd done it numerous times, and each time I called the board's attorney. He told me under no circumstance should I attend those illegally called meetings, otherwise that would make me complicit, and he advised the board not to meet without following all the necessary laws. The board basically ignored him: they felt they could do whatever they wanted to do.

So, unaware of what the board was up to and with the Christmas holidays approaching, John and I got ready to drive to San Diego to see Gary, who was stationed on the aircraft carrier USS Constellation. During our visit John vacillated between having a nice visit with Gary and being so aggressively critical of him that it caused private arguments between John and I. Gary managed to handle it without a serious confrontation with his dad but I stayed on pins and needles throughout the visit.

When we got back, a registered letter was waiting for me at the post office. That letter would change our lives.

I was told to present myself at the February board meeting for "board action regarding my contract." John was furious, outraged and made threats toward the board that I just barely talked him out of acting on. I immediately hired an attorney, who just kept shaking his head when John and I went to see him. "I can't believe this board," he kept saying. "You've done more for this school district in the short time you've been here than anyone else has ever done." By the time we visited the attorney I'd discovered that the board had met in secret and how they'd made the decision to terminate my contract. As I outlined this sorry chain of events to my attorney, he advised me that, if they did indeed terminate my contract, they would be ripe for a wrongful termination suit.

January of 1996 was a difficult month for both John and me. It hurt him so much that my board was treating me with such disrespect, and he felt hopeless and frustrated that he could do nothing to help me. In the six years since the accident I'd learned to recognize the signs that John wasn't taking his meds. However, this time my career was falling to pieces. I was so involved in following my attorney's advice to document the board's behavior, keeping my secretary from twisting the knife in my back, plus keeping the school district staff calm, that I didn't realize he'd stopped again until he was rapidly moving toward a manic episode.

I desperately tried to manage John's tremendous impatience, frustration and explosive temper. Nothing suited him. Nothing pleased him. And nothing was what he wanted it to be. I never knew exactly who he would be when I got home in the evening. He would rant and rave, talking in ways I had never heard him talk and making no sense. He was paranoid, and convinced the board had our home bugged. At times he'd refer to himself in the third person, which really freaked me out. I didn't know his new Colorado doctor well and didn't feel confident that he was even the right doctor for John, but I still tried to get him to go see the doctor. He refused.

As time went by, I continued to ask God for strength to handle whichever person John was that day. It was such a dark time. My personal life was a mess and so was my professional life. And then things got worse.

The board's plan for their February meeting was to place me on administrative leave as they prepared to terminate my contract. They were counting on a typical low turnout by parents and other patrons of the district. However, the board president's wife just could not keep the plans to herself. She did such a good job of broadcasting those plans through her network of friends that on the night of the meeting some three hundred district parents and community members showed up.

Several parents had called me to warn me of the board's intentions. They also assured me that the community would not stand for this, and advised me to move the board meeting location because there would be a standing room-only crowd.

John wasn't one of the people filling the room that night. I knew the meeting would be more than he could bear and asked him not to go. Uncharacteristically, he didn't argue. Maybe it was because he was once again in the depths of depression, when he would often be zoned out, unaware of his surroundings and what was going on. Had he been in his right mind, and as he was prior to the accident, he would never have let me be unsupported, and in turn I would have wanted him by my side.

The parents were right about moving location because, along with the three hundred parents and community members, a full complement of media folks showed up for the meeting, including the major newspaper in Colorado Springs along with all three television stations. Fortunately for me (that night and in future coverage), from the beginning of my tenure as superintendent I'd deliberately cultivated a good relationship with all the local media.

The meeting began without event. The board and I moved through the board's agenda just as we always did. Until the time arrived for the standing agenda item called Patron Forum, which gave the community an opportunity to speak directly to the board about their issues and concerns. Then the board president made a stunning announcement. "Ladies and gentlemen, due to the overwhelming number of people who've signed up to speak, there will be no Forum tonight," he told the throng. "We simply do not have time for everyone to speak."

That announcement was loudly booed and several people jumped up, making it clear they would be speaking, no matter what the board said. So, some 200 people ended up speaking, and their message was the same: the board had better not touch a single hair on our superintendent's head, leave her in her position, otherwise we will take all of you down in a recall election. The board listened with arrogant smirks on their faces. However, they were sufficiently affected to refrain from taking any action on my contract that night.

I was drained by the time I got home, where I found John in a very mellow mood, thanks to the bottle of wine he'd downed while I was gone. "If the board acts the way they've threatened, they are in for a painful surprise" he told me. "The community's going to send them packing like no one ever saw before." Clearly the accident had not messed with his politician's instincts.

He advised me to just remain calm, and to carry on leading the district just as I had been. He was most certainly not his true self but I was so glad to see some shades of that former self. I needed my best friend and at least a little of him was there for me that night. Sadly, the next day that John was once again nowhere in sight. In his place was the stranger I'd been dealing with. He was again restless, withdrawn, overbearing and also prone to manic fits and starts.

The next month the board meeting fell in the middle of spring break. The board chose this meeting to accomplish what they had wanted to do in February, reasoning that the community would be gone on spring break. This time the board president's wife kept her mouth shut so there was no forewarning. John didn't attend this meeting either. "I seriously doubt they'll take any action this soon after the reception they got last time," he told me.

Despite John's prediction, the board went into closed session taking me with them to tell me I was being placed on administrative leave and my contract would be terminated. I was remarkably calm, although probably in shock. I remember asking critical questions and, not finding the board willing to answer most of them, I told them they'd be hearing from my attorney and left. They went back into open session and took the necessary action to put me on leave. As I left, I remember a few of my teachers putting their arms around me and asking if I would be okay. They were furious and some were crying. "I'll be okay, no one has ever died from humiliation," I quipped, even though it felt like a death. The principals later let me know they too wanted to console me after the board's action but, after seeing what had just happened to me, they feared for their own jobs.

I was anxious to get home and tell John what had happened before he saw it on the evening news. "The board won't get away with this," he told me, becoming increasingly manic as he talked. In the end I got him calmed down, but all the time was wondering to myself if I'd entered a parallel universe and hoping I'd wake up the next day with my life back.

With John calmer, I called my attorney, who asked me to meet with him at his office the next day. I finally fell into bed, completely exhausted. John didn't sleep the entire night. (With hindsight I see he was sleeping less and less at that time. That pattern would be followed by a complete crash where he'd sleep for 12 to 16 hours at a stretch.)

The next day the phone rang off the wall with parents, staff and media calling. The community was outraged and assured me that there was no way they were going to sit by and let things go unchecked. They immediately formed a Take Back Our Schools organization and researched recall election requirements. John began to come to life. He was usually the one who answered our phone and was in his element advising the group informally when they called. Once again he could use his expertise. No one knew of his problem and it was only after the campaign had been going for a few months that they began to see that something wasn't quite right with him. From my side, I cautioned him to stay completely out of the community's effort because it could harm my wrongful termination suit. However, he just could not help himself and, though he minimized his involvement to some degree, he did not stop acting as an advisor.

My attorney had told me from the beginning that, while the board president's sexual harassment was clearly wrong, the evidence was not strong enough to do much good for me. On the other hand, the evidence of wrongful termination was overwhelming. "Go with the strongest suit," he advised. So began three months of meetings with my attorney, sometimes with John, sometimes alone. The board would counter my responses with offers to settle out of court, which we refused because they were just ridiculous.

John alternated between being devastated and being intrusive and obnoxious with his advice to my attorney. Several times my attorney had to demand that he cease his involvement if he wanted a good outcome for me. John would then be depressed and have almost nothing to say for days on end, sleeping for long stretches. I was virtually alone in our home. Thank goodness for my strong support base of friends and members of the community. Throughout, I stayed busy, as I continued to teach for the University of Denver as an adjunct instructor. Teaching in their Executive Preparation program saved my sanity. I was also trotted around Colorado speaking to administrator groups as well as the state School Board Association, telling my story and cautioning boards about their behavior in both fiscal and personnel matters.

The speaking engagements really appealed to John. "This is our chance to fight back," he'd tell me. He felt impotent to help me in any big way, but he could help me figure out what to say to the groups. It really perked him up, and at times he seemed normal again as we returned to our mentoring conversations. I was aware that he wasn't taking his medicine but, except for telling him he had to and getting barked back at, I was too tired and devastated to really fight him over it.

I realized several things at this time. One was that he was becoming more and more bizarre in his mood swings, more and more a stranger and I was only seeing even the slightest hint of his former personality emerge once in awhile. The other thing I realized was that he was again job hunting for me. John's close identification with my career was back with a vengeance, and he was a man on a mission even more than he had been when we were thinking of leaving Texas. We had many arguments about it because I was much more resentful of his intrusion than in Texas. I was also very anxious about the legal battle, plus I was depressed. About the only thing we had going for us was the fact that money wasn't an issue. Thank goodness.

Being depressed was new territory for me and I was at a complete loss as to how to deal with it as well as John and the loss of my career. I would cry at the drop of a hat, which was definitely out of character. I would see the big yellow school bus come down the highway bordering our property and just burst into tears. This sent John over the edge, and he would alternate between being as wounded as I was or just so mad he would jump in his truck and be gone for hours. This was absolute rock bottom for me and for the first time before or since I began to think maybe I just needed to end my life.

When that thought crossed my mind I knew I was in big trouble. I immediately called my doctor's office and made an appointment. "Well, no wonder you feel this way," she said when I told her my story. "Look at what you've been through since 1990. Ever gotten counseling or something prescribed?" When I told her there'd only been my one fact-finding session with the psychiatrist in Texas, she asked why. "I just felt that I was supposed to handle it all," I explained. "And I hate anything that makes me feel out of control, I didn't want any kind of tranquilizers or sleeping pills in my body."

My first step was to stop trying to be superwoman, she told me gently. The next step was to cut myself some slack, and third I was to get rid of the guilt over John's illness, as I had nothing to do with it. She explained that, no matter what I did, it would never be enough to make him normal or well. Only he had the power to do that and until he exercised that by taking his medicine and getting psychiatric help nothing would get better for him. I am an intelligent woman and I knew all of that in my head but telling my heart was another matter all together. She sent me home with some Xanax, and for the first time in my life I gave in and took it.

I told John about my visit, and what had prompted it. I was coming to understand that when something was just too overwhelming for him to deal with, he simply disappeared into himself. I have no idea where he went. It was like I could see his body but he was invisible in every other way. His response to my doctor's visit was to disappear. I had felt lonely and vulnerable many times since his accident but I can still remember that moment in crystal-clear detail. I simply felt so alone it was like a living entity always with me.

Never before or since have I experienced such absolute depths of loneliness and vulnerability. I know for certain the depressive side of bipolar is so much worse than what I felt, so in that moment I fully understood why John had been at the point of suicide many times since the accident. The wonder was that he let me talk him out of it each time.

The pain of that kind of depression is not just mental, it is also physical because it is what true hopelessness feels like. We take for granted the ability to continue to hope. Without hope there is nothing left. I suddenly realized that is how John felt most of the time. Continuing to struggle to gain a foothold with debilitating depression and loss of all hope requires the greatest courage. He had shown me that courage repeatedly, and I will never know what it cost him to do so. For all the times he had been mean and ugly to me and everyone else, I cannot overlook the valiant effort he made to keep going day by day.

20
Around the Bend the Water is Calm

The day after my doctor's visit I made my usual morning walk to the back of the property, where there was a dry creek bed with just a small amount of stagnant water at the bottom. Our creek was an overflow from a larger creek that was only full of water at times of great rains, a rare occurrence in the semi-arid climate of Colorado Springs. I'd never, in the year we lived on our ranch, seen any fish in the overflow creek. They probably couldn't have survived with so little water. On this particular morning, we'd had an enormous rain storm the day and night before so the overflow creek was full and flowing at a rapid rate.

When I left the house to make the half-mile walk, John was withdrawn and sitting at his computer. I told him I'd be back shortly and he just nodded. Too depressed to even look up.

When I reached the creek, I sat down on the big rock I'd always meditate on, asking God "Why?" and begging him to reach down and make this all better. As I sat there that morning, I noticed a waterfall had formed where the water entered the creek from the larger one above. Looking down, I was shocked to see four minnows in a whirlpool within the waterfall. They were desperately trying to swim up it. "You're trying to do the impossible," I said out loud.

"You can't get back up that waterfall. What you ought to do is just let go and the water is going to take you down stream and around the bend." Because I could see what they couldn't, I told them it was calm just around the bend. In that instant I made a critical connection and, it was as if God himself had spoken to me. "And that is just what you need to do," He seemed to be saying. "Let go, because everything is going to be just fine around the bend."

When I made that connection with the struggle I could see the minnows having, it was one of those watershed moments when the wonderful thing called hope found its way back into my heart. I just couldn't wait to tell John about my morning awakening at the creek and how much it had lifted my spirits. I walked back to the house eagerly and rushed in to find him still sitting at his computer as if in a daze. Once I'd shared my epiphany with him, he just gave me a blank look and stared at me. "I don't get it" he mumbled. I don't know why I thought I would get a normal response, as he certainly was anything but normal these days. However, my immediate thought was a very sad one. The "real" John would have gotten it. He'd have teased me unmercifully about my "woo woo" experience, but he would have understood.

While I was struggling to deal with my situation on a personal level, the community was working diligently to meet the almost impossible requirements for a recall election. To bring about a recall of an elected official in Colorado, you must have petitions of request signed by two-thirds of those who voted to put the elected officials in office. The school board was elected on staggered terms, so the same voters did not put all of them in office. That alone would have made it hard enough. But when you consider that a significant number of my parents were highly mobile military personnel from the five military bases in and around Colorado Springs, it appeared to be an impossible task. I wished them well, but couldn't imagine they would pull it off. People may complain about their elected officials but seldom, when it comes right down to it, are they willing to go the distance to remove them.

But the people in my community were apparently different. They put their lives on hold and carried petitions door-to-door for about two months. Following the recall requirements, they took their final signed petitions to the election clerk. I was stunned to hear that their petitions had been certified, and a recall election for the first three board members was set for August. Those wonderful people had said they were going to do something about it. And they did!

John was delighted, and as amazed as I was. For the next two months the newspapers ran in-depth articles on the entire issue. Being consistently in the news didn't make me happy, but John felt it was justice because the articles were positive toward me. The slant of many articles was that I was the first female superintendent for the district in an environment of old boy mentality; I had disrupted the old boy way of doing business and they had retaliated. One sympathetic reporter told me she'd gotten in trouble with her own boss because her articles were too friendly toward me.

During the time between being placed on administrative leave and the recall election, John continued to scout out positions for me to apply for, both in and out of state, despite the arguments it continued to cause. John was also busy working on the periphery of the recall effort, despite my demands he stay out of it. "I'm not happy about it, John," I told him. "It is inappropriate." Yet he was really ramping up his manic side and was deaf to anything I said. He was the proverbial loose cannon.

By now I was deep into work with my attorney and his back—and- forth negotiation with the board on my wrongful termination suit. In June the board finally got serious, as their attorney had told them they didn't have a leg to stand on. A wrongful termination case would fall my way, and the expense would be enormous. They promptly offered a settlement that my attorney said was the right number. He explained if I decided to go on with the lawsuit we would win but it would drag on for several years. The decision was mine to make.

I was able to catch John in a fairly stable mood after talking to my attorney. "What do you think?" I asked. We discussed the pros and cons, and I told him I was wounded to the core, hated the publicity, was exhausted and just wanted it behind me. The prospect of dragging it on for years, especially with John's condition deteriorating, was unimaginable to me. He put up a little resistance, telling me he wanted me to get some satisfaction out of "beating the board." But I knew it was really that he wanted that satisfaction, as he felt they had done this to him as much as to me. In the end he could see that I needed to heal and stopped trying to talk me out of settling. By the end of June, the settlement was complete.

Meanwhile, the community was organized and moving toward the August recall election for the first three of the five board members, with the second recall for the remaining two to take place in October. John was still very manic in his behavior and the community was backing him out of their efforts as much as possible. I decided that the only way I could get him out of it was to get him to take some trips with me. I told him I just needed to get away. So we began to take mini trips around the state, even though he didn't like to be away from the action. Finally, the first Election Day arrived. It was apparent to the media by early afternoon that the unusually heavy voting would likely not bode well for the three board members on the ballot. By 9:00 that evening the three had been removed. And they had been voted out by a resounding three to one margin. John was just beside himself, and higher than a kite. I was thrilled but extremely apprehensive that he was being so expansive. He was also drinking very heavily. Those two things together gave me a lot to be concerned about.

He stayed on the manic side of the loop through the second election in October, where the remaining board members were removed, again by a three to one margin. The recall organizers quickly set up an election for a new board and by November of that year the new members had been sworn in.

The new board president and vice president called to ask if I would consider returning as superintendent. Though I knew it would devastate John when he learned of my response, I declined. The only reason I had taken the superintendent's position in the first place was because I believed destiny led me to take it, even when I hadn't wanted the job. I responded to the obvious need, and I did what was necessary. Now it was over, my wounds were deep, and I wasn't sure I ever wanted to be a part of the public school system again.

John mourned with me, falling into yet another deep depression. He would flinch whenever I said I'd probably never again be a school administrator. I am certain, since he had taken such ownership in my role and had mentored me to stretch in my leadership, that he felt the loss just as I did. Being my mentor he likely felt responsible to some extent for my situation. As I always did I worried about the depth of his depression especially during this time. It seemed somehow deeper and more oppressive than it had been before. Each time I left the house I wondered if I would return to find he had finally fulfilled his threats to kill himself. He was again drinking very heavily and sleeping long stretches at a time.

21
Alabama and a New Beginning

Some months after the fact, I was told that the district attorney in Colorado Springs had completed his investigation of the former school board's criminal activity and substantiated their wrongdoing. He explained to the new board that the next step lay in their hands. Namely, the law was such that the decision to prosecute the former board members would reside with the new board. They had briefly discussed this with me when the first three board members were recalled. I didn't try to influence their decision one way or another. I simply reminded them that the district needed to heal, and that the students deserved a district at peace so the focus could return to developing their potential. Whatever would accomplish that should be the only consideration. In the end they apparently decided that the former board president and vice president especially had been thoroughly castigated in the press as well as the community, lost ground in their careers because of it and prosecuting them would not bring the peace I had spoken of and that they all wanted so desperately. They chose not to prosecute. I thought it a very wise decision and certainly made in the right spirit. I long ago found my own way to forgiveness of those old board members, and rarely think of them or of what they did to me.

So, 1996 ended and John had grown much more solitary; talking very little and continuing to drink. He refused to take his meds most of the time and 1997 began in the same way, with him deeply, painfully depressed. Nothing seemed to give him hope, including the cows and horses he loved so dearly. On the other hand, the Xanax had done its job for me and I stopped taking it in the fall of 1996. I was feeling more balanced and, even in the face of John's deepening depression, my emotions were stable. I felt like me again.

I was feeling so much better that I began to think I needed to "get back on the horse" that had bucked me off. That is, I needed to try one more superintendency. I wanted to be the one to decide when I was through, not have a school board decide it for me. I needed to know if I really could go the distance. John didn't comment when I told him. That was quite a surprise as I expected him to be thrilled and set about giving me more help than I wanted. However, he was silent, which gave me pause.

Spring and summer of 1997 was a time of great hopes and of dashed hopes. I prepared my resume and I knew that the cover letter should include a statement of what had happened to me in Colorado Springs. By this time I'd gathered some of the most impressive letters of reference I have ever had from school district employees and the new board members in the district I had just left. The letters made it clear, in ways which would have been inappropriate for me to say in my cover letter, just what had happened. They clearly told how I'd stood up for what was right, and then paid the price. The letters touched my heart. Normally, John would have taken great delight in those letters too but now he barely acknowledged them, so deep was his depression.

Some districts didn't acknowledge my application while others were intrigued and invited me for an interview. When I thought I wasn't a fit I removed my name from consideration, as was my pattern. Once again, as it had when we were planning to leave Texas, that brought John out of his depression long enough for him to express his disagreement. At times he was furious with me and, as always during this extended depressive loop of bipolar, he was irritable and hateful. I held my own, but after what I'd just been through it was getting harder and harder for me to deal with him. I was reaching the point that he was such a stranger I no longer saw any of the person I had loved, and I began to ask myself why I was continuing to stay. I knew part of the answer was that I couldn't figure out how he'd survive without me. In his manic state he'd given large sums of money away to virtual strangers because he felt he was rich beyond measure and money was no issue. My greatest fear was of getting a phone call from him after I'd left telling me he was hungry or homeless or both because he'd given his money away—or worse, someone had taken it from him. I just could not figure out how I would live with that. Those were the times I felt so guilty for even thinking of leaving him without support.

In the throes of those mixed emotions, I vividly recalled the psychiatrist in Texas telling me that John would be better with me than without me, but I would have to decide at what point that wasn't also true for me. That point seemed to be drawing near, as I was slowly coming to believe I couldn't stay married to him much longer.

John was now someone I no longer loved as I had, and he was drinking so heavily I could barely stand to stay in the same house with him. Seven long hard years had gone by since his accident and I had already passed the average number of years a spouse stays with a bipolar disordered person.

Where once there had been love and laughter, friendship and support, and above all the meeting of two minds and hearts, now there was a haunting husk of our shared life. We were strangers facing each other across a chasm. The grinding rhythm of John's depression, his antagonism towards me and our son, his increasingly violent mood swings as he crashed between manic and depressive—it all wore on me beyond endurance. My compassion for this once amazing man and all he was enduring became interlaced with fear, anger (at everyone and everything—John, God, you name it), and guilt as I felt my love diminish and falter. Seven years. It felt like seven decades.

Once again I was asking God, "Why?" While I was sometimes very angry when I asked, sometimes I was just devastated because I couldn't get an answer. I even began asking God why He had left me. "I did the best I could, and tried to do what was right," I told Him in despair. I just couldn't seem to feel His presence any more. I love to read and find solace in the written word, so I found myself haunting bookstores even more than usual as I looked for answers. Besides *An Unquiet Mind,* there were no other books on bipolar disorder at that time. Back then, I would have given anything to read a book written by someone else in my situation so I would know I was not alone; that others had been through this and survived and healed. That would mean I could too. There was no such book.

I did find lots of books that discussed why we are confronted with situations that try our very soul. Some of them propounded extremely conservative religious points of view, believing that punishment was the answer to the question, "Why?" They told me I had done something wrong, and God was on my case. I had grown enough spiritually by this time to completely reject that notion immediately, even though I'd been raised with that very belief. There were other books that were so far out that I couldn't begin to understand what they were talking about. The day I found *The Course in Miracles* was the day I began the spiritual journey that finally brought me to peace with the why question. That book spurred me to look for others that spoke of a similar spiritual path. I began to understand at a far deeper level than ever before what this experience meant-- though it would take me many, many more years to finally find the answer to my question . Only then did I go on to heal.

As is often true when you think you will never get out of the dark night of the soul condition, out of the blue the Universe starts moving the pieces on your chessboard in ways you couldn't possibly have imagined. It happened to me by way of a phone call from my dad, who lived in Anderson, South Carolina. He had always been my rock in the storm. He was not an easy man but he loved me, hard as it was sometimes for him to be comfortable in showing his love.

He was a member of the Greatest Generation written about by Tom Brokaw. Stoic in nature but with a wonderful sense of humor that acted as counterbalance to his type-A personality, he could always get my thinking on the right path. He often started his instructive conversations with, "Damn it, Donna," which I thought were my first and middle names for a long time.

By this time I'd just about had it with bad news, and my dad delivered the knockout punch in telling me he was very ill. I couldn't immediately take it in because he'd always been a virile outdoor-type of man who never seemed to age. Yet on the phone that day he sounded so weak as he described his heart issues. In that instant, I knew what I was going to do. I just knew I wouldn't have him much longer and I wanted to get as close to him as I could so I could see him as often as possible.

With my dad's phone call, my search for a superintendent's position shifted to the Deep South. I talked it over with John, who didn't have much to say because he was depressed, and also because he so loved Colorado he couldn't imagine leaving. I was, however, determined. Finally I was offered a superintendent's position in a school district just outside of Birmingham, Alabama, which was within reasonable driving distance from my dad. The board appeared to be everything the other board was not. They found the stand I had taken in Colorado, and the price I had paid for it, an indication of my character.

John came out of his depression like a giant whale surfacing. He went from deep depression to manic in what seemed like warp speed. Feverishly, he began planning for the move. He accompanied me to Alabama when I went down to sign my contract. There we bought thirteen acres, which already had a barn and was fenced so we would have a place to immediately put our horses. It was beautiful. However, I knew deep in my bones that we would never build a house together on that property. I knew I wouldn't stay with him that long.

The trip from Colorado to Alabama made the trip from Texas to Colorado and the moves within Colorado seem like a walk in the park. John was manic in its worst and highest form. He walked and talked so fast he couldn't finish one sentence before he had interrupted himself to start another. He was furious and scary when I couldn't understand him and he thought I wasn't keeping up. Fear had started to creep in for me while we were in Colorado but it was just a small thing then. It grew on the trip to Alabama and I knew something was about to happen that would be worse than anything that had happened before. There was simply no other way this could end.

I had no idea what the trip to Alabama, which I came to think of as a nightmare trip on steroids, would be like. We had two friends helping us and we each drove a vehicle following John, who was pulling our horse trailer with the three horses. Normally, he was so very careful in every way with our horses and especially when traveling with them. On this trip, however, he was driving well beyond the speed limit across I-40 daringly weaving in and out of traffic. I feared he would have a wreck and kill himself and the horses. Trailering horses is no small task as they have to be walked and watered every four hours. Even in his extreme manic state John did remember that, all credit to him. At each stop, all of us would try to talk to him about his reckless driving and offer to drive his truck with the horse trailer. I did my best to talk him down from his highly agitated state, which had always worked before. He would have none of it. At one point the two guys helping us tried to physically restrain him from getting back in his truck but when he showed real violence they stopped.

The rest of the trip is a blur for me. I just remember my anxiety level was off the charts and I was consumed with the worst kind of fear. We finally arrived at our new property and let the grateful horses out into the lush pasture. John was beginning to wind down a little bit. I tried to talk to this stranger of a husband about the chances he took with all of our lives, those on the highway we had traveled alongside as well as our horses, and he looked at me as if he had no idea what I was talking about. That again proved to me that when he was at the top of the manic loop he had no idea what he was doing and didn't remember it when he was relatively calm again.

22
The Long Good-bye Comes to an End

I knew this Alabama phase of our lives would be my last journey with John, I just didn't know exactly how it would end. He remained in his manic state for quite some time as we started our lives there, working overtime to squeeze himself into my career once again, trying to tell me how to set up my new superintendency. This time around, I pushed him out of my way every time he started to encroach. The guilt I felt in doing so was enormous, but I knew I had to. I'd started my new job at the end of November 1997, as John was on a descent from his extended manic state to one of depression. The uncertainty of his mood swings frayed my nerves almost beyond endurance. Sometimes his descent was relatively slow, sometimes he would make a crash landing from manic to depressive, and sometimes he went from manic to depressive and back to manic in the span of an hour.

We had booked a Christmas trip to Costa Rica prior to leaving Colorado and, though I now dreaded leaving the country with him, we would have lost a great deal of money if we'd canceled. I have no idea why I agreed to make such a trip but I think by then I was simply too exhausted to argue with him. As it turned out, it was one of the worst trips I have ever made. John was a complete mess.

Nothing suited him. He was rude to the airline personnel as well as the hotel staff, which represented a total departure from the real John. Here we were in one of the most beautiful places on earth and he wanted nothing more than to stay in the hotel room and watch TV.

Prior to his accident, we traveled extensively and were great travel companions. He was so curious about other cultures and had lived in Japan during his time in the service. There he learned to speak the language and completely immersed himself in the Japanese culture. That was how he always approached a visit to a new place. He was such fun to travel with, and I always learned from him as he did meticulous research before we left home.

This time there was no sign of that John, which served to confirm to me that the man I'd married was indeed gone for good. My long goodbye was coming to an end. Sad as that made me, I was now relieved to finally understand that there was absolutely nothing more I could do for him. To remain would not serve me at all. My fear of what he might do was greater than ever. I had to leave, and soon.

As 1997 drew to a close I was thankful at least to be happy professionally. The board I served was everything the board in Colorado was not. They were a joy to work for and with, and I was already putting systems, processes and personnel in place that would critically enhance the way we served students. The staff and community were on board as part of the team to see that our students were well served in ways they had not been in the past.

My professional life was in stark contrast to my personal life. I had visited my dad several times in the few weeks since arriving in Alabama and found him steadily declining. It was hard to see. Though I had no way of knowing then, he would leave us in a little over a year.

With work, my dad's ill health, and John's escalating bipolar behavior it seemed like there was always competing pressure for my attention. I was also trying to work out how to leave John while doing my best to ensure that he had the greatest chance to survive on his own. As always the ever-present guilt was weighing on me and I struggled with it. Intellectually, I completely understood that I had no choice but to leave, yet my heart was breaking at the thought of him all alone. John's mental state at the end of 1997 was as fragile as it had ever been. He returned from our trip even more deeply depressed than when we'd left. Then, in the middle of January 1998, we discovered his sister was very ill. John immediately became frantic, packing feverishly to go to Houston to be with her. I remembered again what Dr. McNamara had told me about how bipolar disordered people react to change of any kind but especially changes of great magnitude. John became more and more anxious and fearful as he prepared for his drive. His agitation caused him to snap at me, no matter what I said or did to help him. He was also talking faster and faster, and his movements were rapid and frenzied.

Having just experienced the worst road trip of my life when John and I drove from Colorado to Alabama, I had every reason to fear for him and others on the highway as he now set out for Houston. Yet, no matter how much I begged him not to drive until he could calm down, he was determined to go right then. In fact, he indicated he didn't know what I was talking about when I said he needed to calm down. He was completely unable to see himself as he was. Even though he always told me otherwise, I knew that he had not been taking his medicine since we moved to Alabama.

However, when I asked the same old question this time, his answer was different, as was the tone beneath it. Looking me straight in the eye as he was leaving he said, "No, I am not taking that fucking medicine. I don't need it any more anyway, so don't keep asking me about it!" There was definitely an implied threat in his words--an alarming first in our relationship. His fierce and determined tone told me that if I pressed him, he would become violent. That confirmed my worst fears and I knew then for sure I was in real danger. Up to this point, when he snapped and argued with me, his tone was simply one of frustration, or of someone who hasn't done what they know they should and hopes a good offense is an effective defense. This was completely different. Back in 1990, I'd told the psychiatrist that if John became violent, it would be a deal breaker for me. That statement still held true, and I knew for certain following this encounter I was fast approaching that deal breaking moment.

After John left for Houston, I debated whether to call Gary and ask for his help or to wait and see if it got worse. I foolishly held out hope that it wouldn't be as bad as my intuition was telling me it would be, and that I would be able to handle it after all. Gary knew his father wasn't doing well, but he didn't have all the details. Once again, I made the decision not to share everything at that time. Gary was within a few weeks of getting out of the Navy, and so I opted not to interrupt his life and burden him with what I saw coming until he was out. And what I thought I saw coming was the mother of all manic episodes. If so, there was no doubt that I would be committing John once again.

I also knew that with the new violent undertones I was seeing that there would be no way I could talk him down nor even begin to handle him physically. It was clear that I ran a huge risk of getting hurt, or worse, if I tried. When John returned from Houston at the end of January all of my fears of what was to come were more than confirmed. He was in a full blown manic state. What made this time different was the intensity, as well as his violent speech. He was ready to fight with anyone that got in his way, asked him a question he didn't want to answer, or even looked at him in a way he perceived to be negative. His paranoia was in full force.

He began once again to speak of himself in the third person, as in, "John does not like what you did." He was wheeling and dealing on the Internet, and when I asked him what he was doing he replied that he was setting up what would be lucrative business deals. He would once again be a successful banker and we would have more money than God. I tried to reason with him and get him to stay off of the Internet as I feared he might get himself in deep trouble making deals that lived only in his grandiose illusions. He completely ignored me. I couldn't watch him as closely as he needed to be watched as I was working long hours in my new position while trying to balance my surreal personal life. I remember thinking, if people knew what my life outside the school district was like, they would not believe it. I didn't believe it myself.

By the first week in February 1998 I knew I had run out of time. I had to call Gary. I was now certain I would be committing John again within days and I knew now I couldn't handle it alone this time. When I called, Gary had just gotten back to Texas after leaving the Navy. I have always loved my son better than life itself but never more than in that moment. Although he was trying to get his civilian life started again, he did not hesitate when I asked him to come to Birmingham. "I need you, Gary," I told him. He assured me he would of course be there. "I'll come as fast as I can," he said. "Don't worry, I will be there for you and Dad," he reassured me.

When I told John that Gary was coming for a visit, he was initially happy but soon began making critical comments. "I bet now that Gary's out, he'll have let his hair grow long and look like a hippy," was a favorite. Even after all of this time, it is still unclear to me why John chose to target Gary so negatively. He loved his son deeply and spoke proudly of him to everyone.

I did my best to ignore John's comments because I didn't want to set his temper off now that I knew there was genuine violence just beneath the surface. Sometimes though I couldn't ignore the comments and let loose on him. Where before he had backed down when I challenged him, this time he did not. He almost dared me to keep it up with his facial expression, but never his words.

Gary flew to Birmingham from Dallas on February 12, 1998 and we picked him up at the airport. My stomach was in knots because I had no idea what kind of reception John would give him, but I had a pretty good idea it would not be pleasant. When I saw Gary I was relieved to see that his hair was still short, but he had grown a goatee. I knew that would be enough to give John the opportunity to hassle him and I dreaded what he would say. At first, he seemed glad to see Gary and hugged him. As we left the airport they talked a bit about Gary's Navy experiences, and how happy he was to be out. However, it was only a few minutes before John started in on Gary about his goatee, and he just kept picking at him. To Gary's credit and intelligence he handled his dad very well, not responding in anger and trying to be patient. However, by the time the next day arrived, Gary was out of patience.

I will always believe that when John couldn't incite Gary's temper with his cutting remarks, and thereby provoke a real all-out fight, he turned his attack to me. He knew that would do it for Gary. His remarks to me that day were vicious, and Gary immediately stepped in. "Stop it, Dad—or else," he warned. I watched in horror as the two of them went at each other verbally. I began to cry at the sight of the two of them—my husband and our only child—angrily tearing at each other with their words. Seeing me cry really sent Gary over the edge. Then, just as it appeared the verbal fight was about to turn physical, John shouted in Gary's face, "I'm going into the bedroom to get my gun and I'll blow your head off, Gary!" (Even though I'd removed John's guns while we were in Texas, he'd managed to get them back, and refused point blank to hand them over again.)

With his devastating words still hanging in the air, John quickly turned and stormed out of the living room to get his gun and make good on his threat to kill Gary. There are times in your life when the situation you are dealing with is so unacceptable and unbelievable that for a time you seem to be standing outside your physical body as an observer. That's exactly what happened to me at that moment. As an observer, I was calm and rational. Inside, my emotions were surging.

The one thing that was crystal clear to me in the middle of this madness was that Gary had to get out of the house right then. There was no way I was going to let him stay and be a sitting duck for John when he returned. In retrospect, I don't quite understand why I didn't think it equally critical that I leave with Gary. Over the years, the only plausible answer I've come up with is that I was afraid John would come after Gary if I didn't remain to deter him. I don't remember being frightened for myself, partly because I must have been in shock and partly because, almost instinctively, though I don't know why, somehow I believed that John wouldn't shoot me. I wasn't as sure about Gary. Even if he did shoot me, I was determined he wouldn't get a chance to shoot our son. "Gary, you need to leave. Now," I told him. He did not like leaving me to face John but he knew if he didn't bring help immediately the situation would be much worse. I was relieved when he opened the door and dashed out, telling me he would go next door and call the police. (This was before we all had cell phones.) I was so relieved he was leaving because I knew from seeing TV and newspaper reports that we had the makings of a murder suicide on our hands.

Gary had barely shut the door when John returned, carrying his gun. I could tell the enormity of the threat he had just made had begun to sink in though, and his posture as well as his demeanor were ones of dejection instead of rage.

I walked over to him, put my hand on his arm gently, lowered my voice and softly said, "John, you don't want to kill Gary or me, so give me the gun." I held my hand out and after only a slight hesitation he put the gun in it. I unloaded it, and put the bullets in my pocket. Then I turned to him. "I've known I needed to leave you for quite some time, but I didn't know when that would be," I told him. "Now I do. I am so through with all of this." He stared at me. "You need to get your things, load your truck and go out to the farm. You'll now be living in the RV." Continuing, I finally voiced the words I'd not been quite ready to say until that moment, "I am filing for divorce tomorrow."

During the previous eight years, I had seen the deep sadness of his condition reflected in his eyes many times but as we now stood and looked at each other I saw something I would not have thought possible. I saw sadness in his eyes this time more wrenching and hopeless than ever. I will never be able to forget that as long as I live. Finally John hung his head and, without a word, he nodded in agreement. Slowly he began to gather his things and left the house. I immediately left to go next door and check on Gary just as he was returning to check on me. The police had been called and in a very short time arrived and began asking questions. As John moved toward his truck to leave one of the patrolmen spoke to him, reiterating that he had to leave and should not come back.

So began the aftermath of almost thirty years of a relationship, which had produced a wonderful son and now was broken beyond repair. I couldn't cry any more. I was weary and shock had certainly set in. It felt like I had just witnessed a death. In a way, I guess I had. I remembered again my initial thought after John's accident: that we would all have been better off had he died on top of the mountain in Colorado. That ending would have been far preferable to this one, and to what was to come for John.

On February 14, 1998 I filed for divorce. I realized at that moment that it had been inevitable that his accident would lead me to this moment, given his refusal to manage his condition. When my board members found out what had happened, they could not come quickly enough to offer their support. I will always be grateful to them. Those who could not come personally called to reassure me that they were there to support me. Given how I had been treated by my former board, I was appreciative beyond words. It was my board president who recommended the attorney I hired to handle the divorce.

Now began the long torturous road to dissolving a thirty-year marriage, which until 1990 had been a good one, though not perfect. A marriage not without its problems from time to time but on balance a good one. We had been best friends until the accident and that loss was the worst for me to deal with. I was relieved to have John gone but at the same time it made me remember the good times even more. I am comfortable most times in my own skin but at that moment I felt lonely and very empty. I wished for nothing more than peace.

23
The Divorce and Two More Commitments

Gary left to pack up his things in Texas and move to Alabama, where he planned to find a job and help me. Within a week he was back and had moved in. I will always be grateful to my son for completely changing the original plans he had for his life after getting out of the Navy in order to live with me and help me through such a devastating time. As the days passed, we helped each other with what was a most difficult time in both of our lives. I worried about the very real possibility that John would again confront Gary and threaten his life. "Don't worry, I can handle whatever comes along," he assured me. Although we didn't discuss it, I also know he was not about to leave me to face the aftermath because he feared for my life too.

Within a week or so of filing for divorce, I got a call from a lady who managed a KOA campground just north of Birmingham. She asked if I was Donna Nicholson. "Yes, I am," I said. "And is your husband John Nicholson?" she said as she gave our address. Already my stomach had dropped down to my shoes with dread. The story she told me shows just how bizarre a bipolar disordered person can be when they're in a manic state. It seems John began to drink very heavily after I made him leave and soon found himself again in a full blown manic state. He'd hooked the RV trailer to his truck and driven to this particular KOA. By the time he arrived, it was one in the morning. Of course, the manager now on the other end of my phone line wasn't available, the campground was closed and everyone was asleep.

In his manic state, John wrote a check for $500 and attached a note explaining this was his deposit for a week's stay and asking for the very best space they had. "That's way more than what we charge for a week's stay," the manager told me. Regardless, John placed the check and his note in the night drop box. He then parked both the truck and RV in a spot that wasn't a designated camping space, wedging them between two large trees. "I've no idea how he even got the rig in there, let alone the trailer. That RV looks as if it's never coming out, it's lodged in so tight," she told me. By the time she got on the scene, there was no sign of John. He and his truck were gone.

I knew he was on a manic jag for sure. I just didn't know where he was or how to find him. He needed to be in the hospital but it would be a battle to get him there when we finally found him. I turned to the ex-mayor of the town, who had been so helpful in getting us settled when we arrived. We'd never discussed John's bipolar disorder so when I asked him to help me find John he was surprised to learn about his illness. John was such a great actor when he didn't want anyone to know of his mental issues, so it was natural for the mayor to be shocked and somewhat uneasy initially. However, he did believe me. He and his sons began to speculate on where John might have gone after he left the campground. They got a map of the area and began a search, grid by grid. Their methodical search paid off.

One of the sons found John's truck in the parking lot of a popular Mexican restaurant, saw him inside having lunch, and alerted the police who calmly went into the restaurant and talked to John. They were able to coax him back out to his truck where they cuffed him and took him to Baptist Hospital's psychiatric wing. The mayor told me later when his son found John's truck in front of the

Mexican restaurant the back was filled to overflowing with all kinds of things that John had apparently bought on a spending spree at a convenience store truck stop. There was everything from sports paraphernalia for both the University of Alabama and Auburn to tons of junk food. Nothing John would ever buy in his right mind. It was heartbreaking because some of what he had were things he knew Gary liked to eat and I recognized a few things I liked. Somewhere in his befuddled mind he was thinking about both of us.

The police called me from the hospital as they were admitting John, and it was immediately apparent that he was resisting them with everything he had. I could hear them trying to calm him down and I could hear him fighting back, bellowing every profane word he knew.

I was devastated to realize it had once again come to this—another commitment. After he threatened to kill Gary, and I sent him away, we discussed setting everything in motion to commit him but as obviously out of control as his behavior in threatening to kill Gary was, had we done that, it is highly likely that we would have had to file charges first with the police and jail would have been the consequence, as opposed to committal. I did not want him jailed because I knew he needed treatment—his meds faithfully taken for at least 21 days to get his system balanced. So we chose to give the situation a little time because we knew committing him again was a foregone conclusion. It was just a matter of when the next episode occurred. Now it had.

The guilt I'd felt the first time in committing John came flooding back. I began to second-guess my decision, but I knew in my gut there was no other choice. As I had learned from the previous commitment, when you have to put someone you love in a mental hospital it feels like you have violated that person's basic rights as a human being. It tears at your very soul and leaves an indelible scar.

I was told I needed to contact the county judge, who I knew through the school district functions he attended. "As this is the first time John's been committed in Alabama, you can only commit him for seven days," he explained when I got hold of him. "I'll need to convene a hearing, and I'm happy to hold it in the hospital." I will forever be grateful to the judge for that, otherwise John would have been cuffed and brought to the courthouse by the Sherriff in his official car. I didn't want that for John again. It would be a replay of his first commitment, back in Texas, and I couldn't bear to think about that for his sake—or mine.

After the judge talked to John he asked me if I was sure he was disturbed enough to commit him. By now I was accustomed to this kind of reaction, and calmly explained that John was a consummate actor. "When he doesn't want someone to see his disorder, he has an uncanny knack for hiding it," I told the judge. He looked skeptical, but he respected me so he convened a hearing.

That hearing was just awful. John started out showcasing his acting skills, and appearing completely normal. But as time went by he just couldn't hold it together. He began to raise his voice and shout profanity at all of us, and threaten Gary, the judge and me. The judge gave him a stern warning about his behavior and then continued the hearing. That worked for awhile but in a few minutes he got off on a tangent about how I had lost my faith and didn't even believe in Jesus anymore. No one including me knew where that came from, or why he thought it so important. Through his bizarre behavior he made it easy for the judge to see just how disturbed he really was and he was committed for seven days.

After the hearing I visited with the judge, letting him know once again I was concerned with the length of the commitment. "That's not long enough," I told him. "It will take at least 21 days for John's meds to take effect and calm him down." I had no need to worry, said the judge. "If he's still behaving in a manic way after his release in seven days, he can then be committed a second time—this time for 21 days." I was certain there would have to be a second commitment and I knew then he would be forced to get back on his medicine. That was my only hope. My fear was what he might do when he got out in seven days time.

Gary and I visited John as soon as the psychiatrist told us we could. During those seven days sometimes we could visit with him but sometimes it was impossible because he was just so hostile to both of us.

When John was released toward the end of February he went back to live on our little farm in the RV. Soon he'd begun a campaign to get me back. He began by calling—and he knew just how to hook me. First he told me he was having trouble getting his clothes clean because he had no washer or dryer. "I don't want to go to the washateria in town because everyone looks at me, and I know they're talking about me." I told him I understood. "Bring your clothes here every week," I said. "I'll wash and dry them, and you can pick them up when they're ready." I knew full well what he was doing, but I also didn't want him to be without clean clothes. I was taking a chance that probably wasn't very smart, as I now knew what kind of violence he was capable of. Typical of John's natural need to control which was accelerated by his manic state, he began to complain after a few weeks about how I was folding his things--suggesting ways he preferred them folded. That brought a swift end to my good-hearted offer and I told him I had a perfect solution for that—he could fold them himself so not to bring his laundry back again.

John also began sending a dozen roses to my office every day, with notes begging me to let him come back, to change my mind about a divorce, to please forgive him, and so on. He promised to take his medicine like he was supposed to and to get psychiatric help. He was so sorry he had caused so much trouble for me, he loved me and I would always be his wife no matter what. Saying that this barrage was excruciating would be an understatement: I held my breath everyday when the roses were delivered. I knew I would have to sit him down and tell him there was no possibility that we could ever live together again. Hard as that was going to be, it wasn't the most difficult message I'd have to deliver. It took me a long time to find the words to tell him that I no longer loved him as a wife should love a husband because I didn't know who he was. It was true, but that would make it no less difficult to deliver.

Not long after John began his campaign to get me back, I think Gary became very concerned as he watched me struggle with John's attention and promises. Reflecting on his concern I realize now that he was worried that I would become a victim of my own compassionate nature and take his dad back. He knew that would be a mistake and set out to help me close that door by telling me something he'd kept to himself until now, and that he (correctly) believed would slam the door on John forever.

The evening began without a hint of what was to come. After dinner, as we sat talking, Gary finally told me that his dad had been unfaithful to me. He knew I was going to confront John very soon about his efforts to get me back, and I believe he wanted me to have the complete picture before we met.

The news absolutely knocked me to my knees. Shattered and shocked to my very core, I could not get my mind around what Gary had said. I had never suspected John's betrayal during our marriage.

Gary told me that his dad had engaged in multiple short-term affairs. He didn't know when they had all occurred, just that they had. As he talked, my mind was rapidly flipping through my life with John as if on fast forward, frantically looking for the smoking gun I had obviously missed. I was trying to understand *when* John had his affairs, since there weren't any large amounts of his time that couldn't be accounted for. Of course, I told myself, a cheater would, and could, lie about their whereabouts. There again, he rarely traveled without me, except to a few regional conferences. I attended state conferences twice a year, but he was home with Gary while I was gone. And we spent most of our leisure time together. *When? How? Why?* My mind screamed those three questions over and over and over again.

As I tried to figure out when the affairs happened, I began to wonder if it was possible they were going on even before his accident. After his accident, I reasoned, they must have been during his manic episodes, as I knew when he was in the depressive side of his illness he was zoned out and almost completely inert. I also knew that when taking the full dosage of his meds, intimacy was at best difficult for him. Now Gary's shocking information posed a new potential rationale for his consistent refusal to take his meds.

Regardless of when he was unfaithful, the news was a crushing blow and rocked my world. I felt as if I had been knocked to the ground and just couldn't seem to get up. I began to question both my intelligence as well as my intuition, which has always been keen. How *could* I not have known?

In 1995 when I read *An Unquiet Mind* the author talked about her own promiscuity and risky sexual behavior as a result of her bipolar disorder. (I have since read many research studies that always include promiscuity as a characteristic of bipolar disorder.) At the time, I didn't relate to her behavior because I could see no evidence of it in John. Once I knew John had indeed exhibited this attribute, then I questioned whether he was bipolar all along, or was he just a cheater? This also begged the question, if he was bipolar all along, then was it inherited? That's a question I had asked myself before. The most devastating question of all for me was, if I had known he was unfaithful before I finally began divorce proceedings, would I have stayed with him as long as I did? That was the million dollar question. I spent many heart-searching hours going back and forth, occasionally teary-eyed, more often agonizingly dry-eyed. Once I reached a point of clarity in my thinking I answered my own question: If I had known, I would not have stayed with John as long as I did.

In light of this horrible disclosure I also began to question the authenticity of my marriage and John's love for me. It was an awful time of self-doubt. It is difficult to adequately describe the raging anger and then the grief I felt when I thought about this ultimate betrayal. After all, when we met, I'd had to really stretch to even learn to trust again after my early experience, and it was John who taught me how. Now it felt as if that absolute trust which I'd worked so hard to develop had been thrown back in my face. Besides being husband and wife, John and I had been very close friends for almost thirty years. How does one friend do that to another? Was it purposely done? Was it a result of his bipolar disorder? Did he have an addiction to sex, or was I just not enough? On and on I wrestled with it in my mind. It nearly drove me over the edge, taken along with all of the other drama occurring. I vacillated between wanting to punch his lights out, feeling inadequate as a woman, and grieving the loss of someone I had thought was a faithful husband and friend.

At the height of my pity parties, I finally gave myself a stern lecture. I decided his actions were not about me but about him. If his actions were precipitated by his illness, then I had no problem with extending empathy and understanding, but if he was simply a cheater then I reasoned it still had nothing to do with what I did or didn't do. In that case, it was all about his character. Since I'd seen his strength of character demonstrated many times it was easy for me to believe that wasn't the issue. And after reflecting long and hard on his relationship with me, I believed with all of my heart that I had not been deceived about the depth of his love for me throughout our marriage. There were just too many signs of that love to discount it even now that I knew he'd deceived me. All that said, I struggled with John's infidelity for so many years before I finally came to peace and forgiveness.

One Saturday not long after Gary had shared his devastating news, I asked him to go with me to see John so I could tell him to stop sending the roses and that our marriage was well and truly over. The ride to the farm from the house was a long and anxious one. I knew the hurt I was about to inflict and I knew it would surely send John over the edge. That Gary was willing to go to see his father again after what John had threatened him with the last time they were in the same room still amazes me. (Our son is an amazing person all around, truth be known.) Gary told me he wasn't afraid. We'd taken all of John's guns away once he'd left the house after threatening to kill Gary. It was my board president who suggested that we get them out of the house, and he'd been willing to lock them up in his house. So, as far as we knew, John now had no access to guns.

Shortly after we arrived at the farm he came out of the RV and we sat down in lawn chairs facing each other. "Gary, give us a few minutes alone, would you son? John asked. He acted as if he had never threatened to kill his only child. "Sure, I'll leave you two alone, but I'm not going to be very far away, Gary replied. "I'm warning you, Dad. You need to treat Mom well."

With Gary out of earshot, John started telling me the things he'd said in the notes with the roses. I quickly stopped him. "John, I need for you to understand that your bipolar disorder has made you a stranger to me," I told him. "And refusing to take your medicine and get psychiatric counseling has turned you into someone I don't like, and now fear." I also told him that he, and he alone, had to take responsibility for managing his bipolar condition, and based on what I'd experienced for the last eight years I didn't believe he would ever do that. "There's something else, John," I told him. "I now know about your affairs. Tell me, were they worth it?" As his face froze, I asked him the question that I could not get out of my head, and the only question I really wanted an answer to. "Why, John? Why?"

Clearly caught off guard, John was struggling to speak as the color drained from his face. With tears in my eyes, I told him, "I no longer love you as a wife loves a husband, John. I will always love you as a friend and be concerned for you. I will always hope for the best for you, but I will not live with you anymore." He looked at me with tears in his own eyes and finally his words came as he hung his head. "I am so very sorry for everything, including being unfaithful. And no, it wasn't worth it." He leaned towards me, which made me flinch away. That seemed to shock him, but I couldn't help myself. "I don't know why I did it but, Donna, you're my wife. We've been together a long time and I love you deeply. We are comfortable together. Please don't leave me." I stood up to go and told him this was one of the worst moments in our lives, and one that would likely haunt both of us forever, but there was no other solution. "You need to accept and honor my decision." Then Gary and I left him standing next to his RV looking utterly lost. That conversation lives with me even today and it takes very little to move me right back to that horrible moment.

During this time I worried for and about John's well being and talked to Gary about it. He told me, as he had many times before, "Mom, you can't make this all right for him. He has to take responsibility and he isn't. Yes, he needs help but you need to stay strong and just get through the divorce." I honestly would not have been able to cope with the enormity of it all had it not been for Gary's support.

It wasn't long before we began to hear that John was on a manic high, driving recklessly, drinking and raising hell generally all over the area. Shortly after hearing about his out of control behavior John came to the door one night unexpectedly. Gary was gone and I was alone. I didn't want to let him in but before I could lock the door he pulled it open and stalked into the house. He began to threaten me. He had some kind of alcoholic drink in his hand, and it was obvious it was not his first drink of the night. He was talking a mile a minute and once again interrupting himself as his thoughts were coming so rapidly he couldn't finish a statement before he had another one out of his mouth. Shaking, he stalked through my house, talking ever louder. I realized he had lost a tremendous amount of weight and looked horrible. Even in his rage he looked lost and pathetic. He began to wring his hands and said he was sick, and then switched from threatening me to begging me for help. I had said very little to him until this point but began trying to assure him that I could get him help, but he was going to have to go back to the hospital to get it.

He exploded. "There's no fucking way I am ever going to go back to the hospital again, and you better never even think of committing me again!" I thought he was going to hit me. Still, I looked him straight in the eye and told him to get out of my house and never come back again. By this point I was furious with him and didn't even consider that he could have beaten me to death. He responded by looking like he might do just that, but I never wavered, and my look dared him to argue with me. As I had seen happen many times when he was at the height of a manic episode he suddenly went limp and expressionless--like a balloon that had been stuck with a pin when the air rushes out. He hung his head, said he was sorry, and left the house.

The phone rang. It was the only female board member I had and she was just calling to see how I was. I burst into tears and told her what had just happened. "I'll be right over," she said without hesitation. She called the board president and they both arrived within a few minutes. They were wonderful. They comforted me and asked what they could do to help. After they left Gary came home and I filled him in. We both decided that we had to once again intervene and have John committed. This time it would have to be for the full 21 days so his meds could take effect completely.

I called the judge, who sent the sheriff out to the farm. John was in his RV, drunk and now completely depressed. For the second time I signed all the papers to commit him. Back at Birmingham's Baptist Hospital they once again removed his belt, shoelaces and anything else he could use to kill himself with. Once again the judge held a hearing in the hospital, with Gary and I both present. Once again it was horrifying to watch John. This time though he wasn't hostile. He looked scared to death, shook, and had the same hollow-eyed lost look I'd seen before. It was a wrenching experience for all of us. The judge committed him for a full 21 days. That was the third and last time I had him committed.

As before, sometimes Gary and I would visit and find John civil, and other times we weren't able to stay. One visit is as clear to me today as it was all those years ago. When Gary and I arrived John reminded me of pictures I'd seen of the concentration camp prisoners in World War II. He was shrunken from losing so much weight, the medicine had made him docile and his eyes had a vacant look to them. As I had the other two times he was committed, I asked myself if in fact I really had to do this to him, or had I just over-reacted? The guilt I felt was palpable. His mood ranged from impatient to hostile to clingy and needy during our twenty-minute visit. It was difficult to remember the John prior to the accident, who was so fiercely independent and in charge of his life.

As Gary and I said our goodbyes he stood in the doorway and asked if he could have a hug—just like a lost child. "Of course," I said, and we both hugged him. "John, please never think you are not loved," I told him. You are well loved, we just cannot live with you." We turned and left the hospital. From that moment on no matter how hard I tried, I could not make myself visit him in the hospital ever again. I had reached my limit. It was definitely not an easy decision to make, but I knew I needed to make it for my own well-being. I wouldn't see him again until the day our divorce was final, some seven months later.

When he was released from the hospital after 21 days, I was told he actually looked much better and was calmer. He was stable for the first time in a very long time. I dared to hope that maybe, as he felt so much better, that he would actually continue to take his medicine consistently. I was wrong. Later I learned that he left Birmingham for a while in March and drove to the town where we'd at one time owned a second home in a small private lake community. Some of the best times in our lives as a family were spent at the lake. That's where we met and made lifelong friends with three guys across the lake. One had since died, while the other two were PhD-level health care professionals working in a hospital in town. It was to them that John fled.

The story these two friends tell of John during his stay with them is a classic description of what untreated bipolar disorder does to a life. He parked his RV on their property and hooked up to their utilities. They reported that, at first, they were so glad to see him and talk about old times. John explained that he and I were separated, but they said he reported it was an amicable split. He did tell them he'd had an accident. His warped description of the accident included him actually falling, with his horse, off of the cliff, which he said was five miles below the drop off. In John's version, he fell to the bottom of the cliff and I was left on the top, crying and screaming for help. According to John, a helicopter arrived, took him to the hospital, and that's where he recovered. Our friends said that was among the first inklings they had that he was not in his right mind.

John finally got around to explaining that his sister, who lived in Houston, was back in the hospital and not expected to live. He needed to be within reasonable driving distance in order to visit and ultimately to plan her funeral with her children and that's why he had come to their home, which was a relatively short distance from her. The next morning, he was gone, headed to Houston in his truck, leaving his RV parked on their property. Several days went by, and then our friends got a call from John explaining his sister had passed away, and asking that they watch over his things, as he didn't know when he would get back.

When he finally returned, he went into his RV and remained cloistered there for several days. Neither of our friends thought that unusual, given the loss he'd just suffered. When he came out, he went up to their house with a drink in hand. "Have a drink with me," he said.

The friends said he seemed very jovial, which surprised them given what he had just been through with his sister. As they chatted, John asked if they'd go back with him to Birmingham and help him move some of the remaining things he had at my house and in the barn at the farm. Both guys said at this point there was nothing unusual about John's behavior so they agreed. There had been no mention of negative feelings for me, and in fact they both felt he was still very much in love with me. They had no idea what had actually happened in Birmingham or that he was mentally ill--even though his account of the accident left them with an uneasy feeling. They suspected something wasn't quite right but, again, John the actor had worked hard to hide his condition. As they soon discovered, it would not stay hidden for long.

PART FIVE

LIFE AFTER DIVORCE
THE DRAMA CONTINUES

24
Out of the Hospital and Moving On

As they were packing up to leave for Birmingham both guys were surprised when John told them when they got to Birmingham they had to be careful not to let me see him there. If I did, they had to be careful not to antagonize me or I would have him locked up again. Their feeling was that he was frightened of me and his paranoia was beginning to surface. Both men knew me very well and on the face of it this made no sense. The men demanded to know what was really going on and John admitted he had experienced some temporary mental issues after a fall from his horse on a horse packing trip to Colorado but that his issues were mostly the result of the recent death of his father. He told them because of those very insignificant mental issues I had him committed to a mental hospital.

They said he described this without any sign of resentment. However, when they arrived in Birmingham John became very agitated and displayed ADHD and OCD behavior while his paranoia was in full force. When he realized everything he wanted to retrieve from the barn wouldn't fit in his pickup he rented a U-Haul. They left for the trip back to Texas with the two guys driving the U-Haul and John driving his truck. They reported the trip back was horrible and dangerous. Their descriptions of his fast and reckless driving were a replay of the two moves we had made—Texas to Colorado and Colorado to Alabama. Once they were safely back home they knew it would no longer work for John to stay at their place and tactfully asked him to find somewhere else. John agreed, put most of the stuff he moved from Birmingham in a storage space he rented and arranged for a couple to clean his RV before departing.

Once the couple had finished cleaning, John didn't like how they had done the work and refused to pay them. They called the police and there was quite an altercation with the police demanding that John pay the couple, get out of town and not come back. He did pay up, but had more trouble as he was leaving. He stopped for gas and then became so agitated he just drove off with the gas line still attached to his truck. That further delayed his departure as the police were called and he had to settle the damages. The police then demanded again that he leave town and not return.

As the two guys reflected on the many bizarre and abnormal incidents during his stay with them for this book they remembered several that were hard to believe. Shortly after John arrived at their place following his release from the hospital in Birmingham he invited them to his RV for steaks. He was cooking them on the hibachi outside and when the wind became high he simply put the lit grill under the trailer. When the guys asked him to take it out because it was dangerous he became furious and they began to see the violence coiled just beneath the surface.

One of the most bizarre incidents occurred when John had been away for a few days and they got a call from him. He was in Waco, Texas and had become completely confused about where he was and how to get back to their home. Prior to his accident John had an excellent sense of direction and would never have been at a loss as to how to get from Waco back to the lake. He had traveled all over Texas his entire life, especially the I-35 corridor and east Texas. The guys also remembered that as time went by during his stay he ate less and less and drank more and more. They said he was around 130 pounds, which on someone six feet tall makes them look emaciated. They recalled at times he just had a vacant look on his face as if there was no emotion at all. That is the same look I had seen many times when he disappeared emotionally.

September 17, 1998 arrived and I saw John for the last time. That day my attorney, John, his attorney and I met in Birmingham to finalize our divorce. I had filed in February so it had taken seven months to reach this point. During that time I had John committed twice.

When I saw him in the attorney's office I wanted to just sit down and weep. He looked horrible, gaunt and utterly lost. He was scared to death, he was wringing his hands, and he couldn't seem to get his words out. He was so fragile.

I had already told my attorney that, even though Alabama was not a community property state, I wanted everything to be split as equitably as possible. We had many assets that I would need to liquidate but when I had done so the proceeds would be split equally. I further insisted that John leave the marriage without any debt. We had very little debt but I wanted to assume what we had. I asked that he leave with his truck and RV free and clear and I wanted to pay for two years of his auto and health insurance

In Alabama, as the spouse with a job, I was required to pay alimony, which I voluntarily agreed to pay at a much higher monthly rate than the court stipulated. I required that he apply for his social security disability within two years and then the alimony would be cut to half that amount a month. He steadfastly refused to even consider seriously pursuing his social security disability, which did not surprise me. It reflected his consistent refusal to accept his traumatic brain injury and his mental illness largely because that was so out of balance with his self image. (I have also learned through more research that bipolar disordered people almost always have no insight into themselves and their illness. They do not have the ability to see themselves as they are.) I further stipulated that all of our investments would be split equally. The most critical requirement for John in our settlement was that within two months he had to leave the state of Alabama and not to return to live there as long as I lived in the state. I had no intention of living my life looking over my shoulder to see if he was stalking me.

That's what my attorney was prepared to offer as the final meeting began. I can only assume that John had warned his attorney that I was somebody to reckon with and that I would fight everything he wanted. I know for certain he had told his attorney that when things didn't go my way I'd had him committed multiple times to a mental hospital.

His attorney immediately began the conversation by threatening me. Before my attorney could open his mouth I abruptly stood up, almost knocking over my chair, and leaned across the table to get closer to John's attorney. "I will not tolerate being treated with anything other than the respect I deserve," I told him. "If you would close your mouth and open your eyes you'd see that I've been more than fair with what I am willing to do for your client." The room got silent. John looked like he wanted to run out the door and both attorneys were shocked. My attorney recovered first and began to describe the terms we had discussed. It did not take long to get to closure of the meeting.

My last sight of John Nicholson was as he walked out the door hunched over and looking for all the world as if he were at the end of his rope. His attorney cleared me a wide path, saying nothing to me as he left. I bid my attorney goodbye and as I left the building I was just numb.

Driving home I reflected on what had just happened as well as what had happened over the past eight years. What had lasted for almost thirty years had ended in under an hour. The man I had fallen in love with, married, had a son with and grown to love as my best friend had actually died on top of the mountain in Colorado in 1990. The fact was, I sent my husband up that mountain but he never came back. Instead a stranger came home to me. A stranger who grew more so daily and who I came to fear.

I could not have known then that, while we were no longer legally bound to each other, the twists and turns of John's life post divorce would not free me by a long shot.

Within a month of the divorce I was deep into the intense drama of liquidating the property assets John and I had. I spoke to real estate agents in Colorado Springs and in Jackson about putting our homes and property on the market. For that, I needed John's signature and finding him was like trying to locate the proverbial needle in a haystack.

He had agreed during our divorce settlement to cooperate with me but now he was dodging contact. He changed his cell number and I had no way to reach him. Within two months he was living in Arizona. I sent letters to his last known P.O. box in Arizona and the letters were returned. I contacted his niece in Houston as he stayed in touch with her. She tried to reach him and was sometimes successful and sometimes not. When she was successful, I would extract a promise from him to phone in on closings when we had a buyer but at the last minute he would not show up. The buyer would walk away and the process would start all over again.

I remember one particular time when he didn't show for closing, and the buyers said they'd sue. They didn't, thank goodness.

John was so manic during this time that there was no telling where he was or what he was doing. I only knew he was avoiding contact purposely. My days were filled with wondering if I would ever walk out from under the ominous black cloud that seemed to have positioned itself over my life and refused to budge no matter what I did.

I discovered that when you can't find someone and you are trying to sell jointly-owned property you can advertise for a specified amount of time in newspapers where you think the missing person might be. If they do not respond in a given period of time, which varies by state, you can petition the court to go ahead and let you sell the property as one of the owners. I was finally forced to do just that. When John discovered what I had done he was furious and blamed me because the amount the property was sold for did not meet his standards. The fact was, the prices were very good and reflected market value. As I had stipulated in the divorce settlement, my attorney always sent him his half of the proceeds. Liquidating our total assets took me about two years because he was manic and totally uncooperative. That was two years of the worst kind of hell.

25
Suicide: The Final Solution

From February until the end of 1998 I was often able to visit my dad in Anderson, South Carolina. He was upset when he learned that John was not doing well, that he had threatened Gary and that I was afraid of him. He, of course, knew that I had committed John three times and he knew about the divorce. He and John had always gotten along and my dad was a great supporter of his. He thought John was very smart and respected his ability as a banker. However, he was greatly relieved when the divorce was final, given the circumstances. By then his health was rapidly failing.

In March I began to plan for the house I wanted to build on the farm John and I had bought. The horses were still there and Gary and I were taking good care of them.

I had long conversations with my dad about the building plans for my new home—he had been a builder and developer, so he gave me good advice. One of the last things he did with me before his death was to walk the area where I wanted to build.

I planned to clear about two acres in the middle of the woods just behind the pastures and barn, and had collected pictures of the many features I wanted in a scrapbook. It was part of my great escape from all the trauma going on in my life. I felt a desperate need for something hopeful to help deal with the enormous distress of John's last two commitments as well as the divorce and difficult process of liquidating our assets. I had lost so much, and I just needed to add some joy back to begin filling the looming void.

My dad approved of the location for the house and made some wise suggestions. When I showed him the initial plans and pointed out that I could "see" a rocking chair with him in it on my porch he looked at me sadly. "I don't think you see me, Donna." He was right. He was obviously sliding downhill quickly, and his once vigorous physical presence was steadily being replaced by a frail, shrunken version.

As 1998 ended, I finished the year busily making plans to break ground for my new home in June of 1999. I spent New Year's Eve with my dad, enjoying two wonderful hours alone laughing and reliving precious family memories. He told me how much he loved both my brother and me. It was very rare to hear him talk with such emotion. In turn, I had a final chance to tell him how much I loved him and how great an influence he'd had on my life. I am so grateful I had that priceless opportunity to tell him goodbye. When I left the next day, as I reached out to gather him in for a last hug, I knew I would not see him again on this earth. Normally, when he bid me goodbye from the porch he would go back into the house before I drove out of the driveway. This time he stayed on the porch and the last view I ever had of him was from my rearview mirror. I watched him waving goodbye as I drove away until he faded from view.

On January 12, 1999, two days before my dad's 81st birthday, I was leaving a Rotary Club meeting at 1 p.m. Central Time. Walking to my car I suddenly felt as if I had lost all substance and was just floating. I had felt fine all day and can't really say I felt sick, I just didn't feel as if all of me was present. When I tried to open the car door I had to reach for it several times before I connected with the handle. I was badly shaken by this and called my administrative assistant. I told her I was feeling very strange and was going home to lie down for a few minutes before returning to the office.

About an hour later I drove back to the office still feeling not completely present. When I got home that evening there was a message on my answering machine from my dad's wife asking me to call her. I immediately knew my dad was gone. The way I had been feeling all afternoon now made sense. I called her and learned that my dad had indeed passed away of a massive heart attack. "When?" I asked. "It was at 2 p.m. Eastern Standard Time," she said, which of course was when I was leaving the Rotary Club. I now know the sensations I felt leaving the meeting were due to what is known as a shared death experience.

Somehow John was told of my dad's death and a few weeks later I got a very sweet card from him letting me know how sorry he was. He described the immense respect he had for my dad and his own personal sorrow at his death. In the card he expressed his understanding of how hard this would be for me to deal with. It made me cry as I realized that, for a brief moment, he was completely aware of what happened and had reached out to me as the John of old would have done had he been with me.

My one intention was now to build my home in the seclusion of my farm and just find peace and healing. The previous eight years, with the trauma of John's accident and resulting traumatic brain injury as well as his bipolar disorder, the devastating experience of my first superintendency and now my knowledge of John's betrayal as well as my father's death, had taken their toll and I was so very weary of spirit and soul. However, there was to be no peace for me.

Several times during the summer and fall of 1999 I received calls in the middle of the night from Arizona highway patrolmen asking if I was Donna Nicholson and if my husband was John Nicholson. I corrected them each time, explaining that he was now my ex-husband. The stories they told me were always variations on a theme. John was driving dangerously fast while drunk on the interstate and had a wreck. It always amazed me that no one was hurt in those wrecks.

As part of my need to ensure the accuracy of this book as I was writing it, I revisited my personal journals and other critical documentation and I discovered John's arrest records. I'd not read them before, and doing so even after such a period of time had passed was difficult. The 1999 arrest records paint a picture of someone totally out of control and who was manic to the extreme. His actions demonstrated his lack of insight, grandiose view of himself, his rage and abject frustration.

In one of the records, the events leading up to his arrest for shoplifting were described. The account shows that he believed he was to be obeyed without question and that he was in control of everything. He had gone into a convenience store with his checkbook in hand, selected two cans of Pringles potato chips, which he proceeded to open and eat before he paid for them as he continued to browse for other items to purchase. As he approached the checkout area he forcefully threw his checkbook on the counter and ordered the clerk—with a profanity-laced command—to fill out his check with the amount of his purchase. He then told the clerk that he would be back in a couple of hours to sign it. She informed him that, while she would be happy to help him complete his check, he could not leave before he signed it. At that, he basically told her he could do whatever the fuck he wanted to, and she could not stop him.

That said he walked out the door, leaving his unsigned check and checkbook with the clerk, got in his truck and peeled out of the parking area at high speed. There was a police car not far away and the cops began to chase him, finally apprehending and arresting him after several blocks. He was taken to jail and bonded out. When his case came before the court he didn't show up, which had become his pattern. I wept for the lost soul John had become as I read the many arrest accounts in those files.

One of the calls to me from the Arizona highway patrol reported that John had picked up a hitchhiker whom he turned his truck and keys over to when they stopped for the night and asked him to go to the store to buy toothpaste as he didn't have any. Of course, the hitchhiker stole his truck. During this year he was also arrested many times for DUI and refused to appear in court. He was also arrested for running red lights and harassing as well as threatening people. Warrants for his arrest were posted and somehow he was always able to elude their efforts to catch him

I questioned the patrolmen about why they kept calling me, since John was my ex and I had nothing to do with his life anymore. Each time they responded that John had pleaded with them to call me because I was his wife and I was the only one who could really help him. Though it devastated me to hear that, I knew that I had to resist getting pulled back into his nightmare. Guilt was my constant companion but I stuck to my guns. The price I paid was constantly being in a state of dread, particularly when my phone rang late at night. To this day I do not know how I survived that time in my life and continued to function. And I fully understand that as true as that is, John was so much worse off. He was utterly lost and seemed not to be able to find his way out. Who would have ever thought that our promising beginning as husband and wife would lead us to this?

At one point during the year my attorney called me to say he had gotten a call from John who had been badly burned in an accident. For some reason he was clearing land and had poured kerosene on a pile of brush. The fire got away from him because, I suspect, he was drunk. He called because he had lost his insurance card and needed the information for treatment.

The arrest records make it clear that John's actions that year, especially from August through early November of 1999, were those of someone who repeatedly violated the law, engaged in risky behavior, was arrested, did not show up for court hearings and believed he was above any law. He was clearly on a course of self-destruction. In the first week of November all of John's issues with the Arizona police and highway patrol reached a critical point. The penalty when he could be apprehended was to be six months in prison.

Finally, he was picked up. He was taken to jail and once again bonded out. (Why they kept letting him bond out when they knew his pattern of not showing up for his hearings is beyond me.) However, this time when he did not show up it was because he fled the state. An arrest warrant was immediately issued as well as an all-points bulletin. This time they intended to apprehend him and they had no intention of letting him out of their sight until he had been remanded to prison. John knew his time was up. He also knew the consequences for his actions and choices would be extended time in prison. I suspect he was weary of running and very depressed, but the thought of being imprisoned propelled him to run one last time. He intended to make it his final act in this tragic drama.

In the pre-dawn hours of November 9, 1999, nine years almost to the day since his first manic episode, which had resulted in his first psychiatric commitment, as well as two weeks prior to what would have been our 31st wedding anniversary, John traveled alone east on I-40, crossing from Arizona into New Mexico. At some point that morning he exited I-40 and made the fateful turn onto the Zuni Indian Reservation.

His intention was clear—to kill himself and thereby be released from the tangled mess he had made of his life as well as the suffocating, black depression.

Pulling to a stop in an uninhabited part of the reservation, he reached across the seat to pick up his .45. He put it under his chin. He had stuffed his front shirt pocket full of newspaper clippings, which told the story of his successes. I am convinced that in his mind he believed that whoever found his dead body would also read the clippings and understand that he had been someone of value and worth. The clippings told the story of what he had been. Now he was dealing with what he had become. He pulled back on the trigger. He exerted the pressure necessary to free the bullet from the chamber and shot himself.

Incredibly, he did not die. We later learned that the bullet traveled through the cognitive areas of his brain, knocking out his teeth, and exiting the top of his head.

He must have been knocked unconscious immediately.

At some point, he regained consciousness and, though it defies explanation, he drove to the small town of Zuni. Witnesses said he parked the rig in front of the hardware store and stayed in the truck for a while. He seemed to be wiping something up, which was of course his blood, as he was bleeding profusely.

With blood streaming down his face, he walked across the street to a restaurant. Though with his teeth gone it must have been difficult for him to talk or be understood, he asked to order something. The owner realized he needed medical attention and called the Zuni police, who called for an ambulance. Once the ambulance picked him up and he was delivered to the Zuni hospital it was clear to the doctors there that they did not have the means to treat his wound. It was obviously life threatening.

The official Zuni police account of what they witnessed when they picked John up at the Zuni restaurant describes a man, dazed and disoriented with an obvious wound in the top of his head and his jaw, who was losing dangerous amounts of blood. When they questioned him the answer he gave says it all. In his now garbled speech he told them he had run into a wall.

The Zuni hospital made arrangements for John to be admitted to the hospital at the University of New Mexico at Albuquerque and called for Life Flight. His identification was in his truck in Zuni, which had been impounded. Apparently no one thought to give it to the doctor and nurse accompanying the flight, nor did they ask for it. I can only assume when he was picked up the urgency to get him to Albuquerque superseded the necessity to know who they were transporting. Thus he became John Doe.

A week later I would receive an unexpected call and the information delivered would suck Gary and me back into yet another chapter in this never-ending drama with John.

26
Recovery

A week after John was delivered by life flight to the hospital at the University of New Mexico at Albuquerque, and while still in a coma, I received a call from the neurosurgeon treating him. John had remained unidentified until someone thought to check with the Zuni police who had removed his brief case, which was in his truck, and contained his driver's license. John's personal belongings were finally sent to the hospital. There was correspondence in his brief-case which led them to one of John's nieces in Houston. She directed the doctor, who was looking for medical history, to me. I told her about everything, including his bipolar disorder, traumatic brain injury and other mental issues. I also told her about his sensitivity to medication. It was a replay of all of the other times since his accident that I'd supplied his medical history to doctors.

The neurosurgeon told me John was in a coma because they believed he had shot himself. When I asked about the prognosis she said they did not yet know because there was so much swelling in his brain it was impossible to determine the extent of the damage done. And, of course, she had not been able to talk to him yet. She warned me that as a worst case scenario he might die, or he might not come out of the coma. Even if he did, he could be mentally impaired beyond his capability to care for himself. I immediately had a flashback to the hospital in Texas when Dr. McNamara told me the medicine he had been given had made John toxic and he might not make it.

I was shaking off those old memories when the Albuquerque neurosurgeon posed a question that might have seemed strange to an observer but not to me. "Do you have any idea why John would pick the Zuni Indian reservation to kill himself?" she asked. "I surely do," I replied. It made complete sense if you understood that all of his life he had been a student of western history, particularly that of the Native Americans. John was of Cherokee ancestry. One of the first books he gave me to read after we were married was *Bury My Heart at Wounded Knee* by Dee Brown. He had an almost mystical connection with the struggle of the Native Americans and always championed their cause.

The doctor promised to keep me informed of John's condition. I hung up the phone and thought of all the times I had talked John out of killing himself and the times he struggled to describe to me what the depression—so black and so oppressive—was like. In frustration, he would always end up saying, "There is just no way I can explain how this depression feels. There is no way you can understand what this is like. I just want to make it stop." Now he had finally followed through with his threat to make it go away once and forever, and still could not find an end to it. I grieved for what depths of anguish and desperation he had to have reached to finally pull the trigger. I wept for the fact that he must have felt unloved, uncared for and so completely alone that he would choose death over continuing his life in this condition. Then I got mad.

I was furious with the God that could let someone so intelligent and gifted, who had so much more to contribute, end up like that. In my anger, as I had so many times in the past nine years, I demanded to know: "Why?" This time I screamed the question at the top of my lungs. I received only silence in answer. I begged God to help me understand, to give me the wisdom to accept this and to find peace. I begged that John be given the same, if he lived. In that moment of tragedy and despair I had forgotten all about the experience with the minnows and God speaking to me through that to tell me just around the bend the waters would be calm. At that moment they were anything but calm. I eventually got my answer and the peace I was desperate for but it didn't come that day. I understand now that I wasn't quite ready for the answer then. I also believe John left this earth without ever finding the answer or finding peace.

In trying to reconstruct what happened to John as a result of his self-inflicted gunshot, I finally found the courage while writing this book to read the reports from the doctors treating him and I found them devastating, enlightening and yet puzzling. After a week in a coma in Albuquerque, as he regained consciousness, the doctors began to question him in order to get a clearer picture of what had happened. John eventually amended his explanation of running into a wall in his truck and told the doctors that someone came to the driver's side window and shot him through the open wing of the window. He couldn't tell them who or give a description of the person. His medical records also reported that anytime the doctors or therapists asked him if he had shot himself he flew into a rage, screaming and shouting profanely that he most certainly did not shoot himself.

They also asked him about his consumption of alcohol, to which he answered that he was only an occasional social drinker and had never gotten a DUI. Actually he had gotten several DUIs after his accident.

The doctors' reports indicate that there was an exit wound in his jaw as well as the top of his head. However, the only bullet hole in the truck was in the top of the cab. The two exit points would seem to be impossible unless the bullet somehow split. However, it isn't likely we will ever solve that mystery and know exactly what happened.

The hospital reports also described, as we already knew, that when he shot himself the bullet had knocked out his teeth as it traveled through his head. As a result he ended up with dysarthria, which is a motor speech disorder. The consequence was a pattern of speech similar to that of stroke victims, as well as intense drooling. Now when he spoke, he did so in a slurred manner and very slowly and deliberately. He displayed limited tongue and jaw movement and initially the reports indicated he had his jaw wired. He weighed 180 pounds when he was admitted to the hospital and weighed 130 when he was discharged several months later, looking gaunt and vacant. During this time, according to the doctors' reports, they had him on suicide watch. Of all of the things for which I am grateful I am most grateful that I never saw John in that condition. I fear that would truly have finished me off. Unfortunately, Gary did see him.

I realized after talking with the surgeon in New Mexico that I needed to call Gary and let him know what had happened and to fly him out to Albuquerque. I called Gary, and he said of course he would go out to help his dad. When he arrived, he found quite a mess. In addition to having to deal with his father's physical condition he also had to deal with his dad's girlfriend. Somehow she'd learned of John's attempted suicide and his hospitalization. She'd immediately made her way from her home in Texas to John's bedside. By the time Gary arrived she had gotten a temporary power of attorney and made fast friends with one of the nurses, who had given her John's confidential records.

Gary immediately protested, as John's nearest blood relative. As ludicrous as it was that Gary should even need to contest his dad's girlfriend's power of attorney, it seems there is a provision for such a scenario in the state of New Mexico. It was imperative that Gary secure the right to make decisions for his father in the very likely event that John would not recover enough to take care of himself. Gary knew if that happened he would need to make arrangements for his dad. (In such an event, our plan was to take John back to the VA hospital in Houston where he would be near his niece and nearer to Gary.)

The hospital convened a meeting to try and settle the matter. John's girlfriend hired an attorney and I hired one for Gary. In the end the hospital decided they would defer the decision to a judge and a new hearing date was set. When the hearing before the judge was held he determined that a management company would take over and manage all of John's rehabilitation as well as his financial affairs until such time as he could function on his own. That settled it.

After John was dismissed from the hospital and it was clear that he would be able to care for himself our attorney told us we had a very strong case for suing the hospital on the confidential records issue. Gary and I discussed it, but in the end we determined that we had had enough. Though we were relieved for John's sake that he would be able to continue living on his own caring for himself, this latest event in our lives had left us feeling broken and so sad. Our goal was to find peace and we knew fighting with the hospital through the courts, given the time it would take to reach a conclusion, would not provide that.

1999 ended with John recovering from his self-inflicted wound. According to the surgeon he had in effect given himself a frontal lobotomy and he would never again experience the manic side of his bipolar disorder. He was now unipolar and would forever be in a depressive state. That was in many ways the cruelest fate of all since it was that depressive state he fought so very hard and hated so much. Now he would be that way until the day he died. With the gunshot he had ended the aggressive state he would evidence when manic and became much more docile.

Looking back, it is obvious to both Gary and me that even in John's downgraded mental state he retained so much of his intellect. To our amazement, we discovered much later that, after he was released from the hospital in Albuquerque, he wrote his life story. Although we found it on his laptop after his death we were too emotional to read it then. Reading it recently as we were doing research for this book it is a testament to his resilience. Surprisingly, his writing hung together chronologically in most places, given the residual effects of his wound. The details of his life's story are distorted in places and it is easy to see how much his memory was gone and at best sometimes unrealistic. But on balance it was compelling writing, and, knowing him as I did, it made me laugh that he had interjected so much humor in his writing even in his by then constant depressive state.

27
Grief

After John's attempted suicide and the struggle his recovery became, Gary and I were desperate for our lives to return to some kind of normalcy. He flew back to Alabama from Albuquerque and returned to work and, as I was still on a quest for peace and some measure of happiness, I turned with renewed energy and joy to overseeing the completion of my new home. The plans had been completed in early 1999 and it then took from June to December of that year to actually build it.

As described earlier, my life after the divorce continued to consist of one devastating challenge after another. I dealt with the many disturbing calls from the Arizona highway patrol and police due to John's continued manic rampage through Arizona and his flight from the law. I had also almost completed the long frustrating process of liquidating our assets without being able to find John for his assistance. And I had just lived through the horror of his attempted suicide as well as the aftermath. While all of this was going on, I somehow managed to retain my ability to fulfill my duties as a superintendent, successfully leading my district through enormous yet necessary changes. My administrative assistant knew the details of what I was dealing with but most people in the district did not.

As I had in Texas after the accident, I was trying so hard to prevent my personal problems from interfering with the positive path the district was on to serve children. Sometimes I wasn't sure if I could do that even one more minute because I was still trying to avoid the crippling emotions I had yet to let surface, and which were getting harder and harder to push away.

So I was exhausted but excited on December 16, 1999 when I finally moved into my beautiful new home. I'd loved every minute of the building process, and it was the one thing in the midst of all of the craziness of what passed for my life at the time that—besides Gary—brought me joy. When I moved in I felt such a sense of accomplishment and hope. John had always been in charge of building our homes during our marriage, even though I had input, but I had built this one all by myself.

Unfortunately, those good feelings did not last long. Over the next week, once I settled in and had everything in its designated place, I experienced an overwhelming let-down. I don't think I realized it would happen yet, once I thought it through, I knew exactly why I felt that way.

I had known all along that building my house was a tactic to avoid the deep grieving which was long overdue. It will be difficult for anyone who has not experienced what I went though or something similar to understand just how critical it was for me to begin adding things back into my life, such as building my home, to counter the many losses I'd experienced over the past ten years. I felt at times that my very survival depended on finding ways to bring joy back into my life.

However, now that the building process was over, I had no place or reason to run from the grief I had yet to explore to its greatest depth. It was stalking me and could not be ignored nor delayed any longer. I would now have to tend to my emotional unfinished business. I know now as I knew then that it is impossible to avoid grief. It can be delayed but sooner or later all of the stages of grief have to be experienced in order to also experience healing and peace.

I needed to stop running from the grief, which was bubbling just beneath the surface.

I had cried during the now ten years after John's accident, and sometimes I'd cried hard, but I never had really allowed myself to feel the absolute depth of the grief I was holding back so tightly. Now, with the house completed, I had no choice but to deal with the wall of emotion that was threatening to overcome me. I needed to finish once and for all my grieving for the humiliating and devastating professional experience in Colorado. I had to finish my grieving for my dad and for the accident that took John from me. I also desperately needed to cleanse myself of John's betrayal of me and our marriage so I could get past the pain to forgiveness. Even after our divorce, and though John was then physically absent from my life, I still held my emotions back but by then it was to protect myself not John. I felt the minute I gave into them I would fracture into a million pieces. And I feared I wouldn't be able to put all of those pieces back together again.

That enormous wall of emotion finally came crashing down on me one cold Friday evening in January of 2000. My administrative assistant came by my house with something for me to sign and, being the wonderful and compassionate friend she was and is, she knew immediately that I was hurting emotionally more than usual. She asked me when I was going to stop holding in everything I had been through and just give myself permission to really grieve the loss of John and our life. "If you had a friend going through something like this, what would you tell that friend?" she asked. I said I would encourage my friend to just let it all go. "Well, I'm your friend and that is what I am telling you to do," came her reply. As tears rolled down my face, I promised her I would do the emotional work that had been delayed for far too long. With a hug and kind words of support she left, reminding me she was only a few minutes away if I needed her. But I knew what I had to do was going to have to be a solitary journey.

After she'd gone, I sat quietly in my new home looking at the flames in my beautiful rock fireplace dancing in front of me until I could no longer see them for the tears falling. I asked God to help me let it all go because I simply didn't know how or where to start that frightening process. With my prayer said, I took a deep breath and finally just let it all go.

Ten years of pent up sorrow fell like rain. Then came great racking sobs. I thought about the loss of my husband—my best friend, my mentor and the person who could always make me laugh with his dry wit. I gave myself permission to feel the absolute depths of the hurt the knowledge of his affairs had brought me. I also thought about the tragedy of John's life and his hurt. I thought about Gary's loss, and the grief he had yet to let himself feel. I mourned the absence of my father and I thoroughly licked my professional wounds.

I forgave myself for the pity party I was hosting in order to begin to heal, really heal once and for all. The depth of my grief fueled my sobs from Friday night to sometime in the wee hours of Sunday morning. My face was swollen and my eyes fire engine red but I was empty. I knew the day would come sometime in the future when I could think of the past ten years from a healed perspective and that brought me great comfort.

Anyone who has ever engaged in the grieving process knows that there comes a point when, even though you feel wrung out with it, what follows is a feeling of cleansing and peace. That is what I felt that Sunday morning. The beginnings of peace and healing had been a long time coming and the road there had been a winding, discouraging and dark one. I knew I still had work to do to finally find the lasting peace and healing I would need but I had at least begun the critical process. I was now able to sleep for the rest of the day—the kind of restorative sleep that also heals. At last I could finally begin to find my way to absolute forgiveness and to moving on.

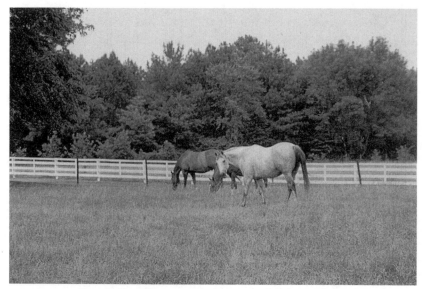

Skip, Red and Dynamite on Donna's Alabama farm.

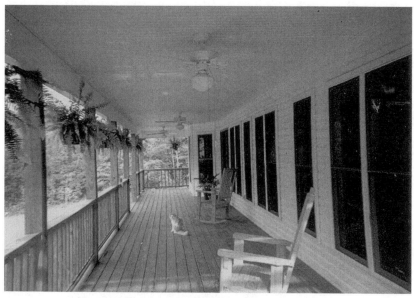

The covered porch of Donna's new home in Alabama
and the rocker her dad never got to use.

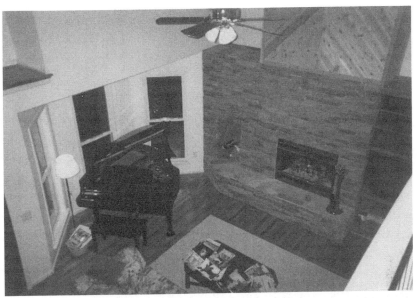

The rock fireplace in Donna's new home.

28
John's Death

O nce John recovered from his wounds and was discharged in 2000 he traveled a little but finally settled in an RV park in Las Cruces, New Mexico. Quite a depressing place actually. He bore the unmistakable results of his attempted suicide. His mental condition made him slower to respond and his physical demeanor made it obvious that something was not quite right. Apparently he lived quietly, heading into town once a week to a nice restaurant for his favorite meal—steak and baked potato. We were told he had red wine with his meal, which makes sense as he was quite knowledgeable about fine wines and preferred the reds. We shared such a meal so many times in our lives together but now his meals were solitary. John never again contacted or spoke to Gary or me.

The evening of January 18, 2004 I received the call I had expected for some time. When I answered, John's niece calmly told me that her uncle had died of a massive heart attack an hour or so earlier. It seems the shower in the bathroom in his RV was not working so he had walked down to the community shower that afternoon. He had disrobed and made it into the shower stall.

It appeared that once in the shower he had the heart attack and had fallen to the floor. He was still alive, but barely, when he was found. An ambulance was called and, as he was being taken to the hospital, they said he was fighting to talk but then simply gave up and slipped away. He was DOA when they reached the hospital. It was just days after his 62nd birthday.

I received the news with resignation and, frankly, relief. I hoped that his tormented soul was finally at peace after thirteen years of suffering the tortures of the damned. What did I feel? The same thing I'd felt so often in the years since his life-altering accident—numbness.

In the years after John's accident I had begun to put together the pieces of the answer to "Why?" The answer helped me in critical ways as it represented a new system of beliefs quite different from that I had grown up with. My new beliefs helped me frame John's death and all that we had been through within the bigger context of the Universe and our real purpose on this planet.

I had now become decidedly more spiritual than religious because of my experiences. And while for me that truth represents tremendous spiritual growth, which I celebrate and am grateful for, I understood quickly that some of my acquaintances and friends who still retained a more conservative religious orientation found my beliefs unacceptable. I understand that everyone has a complete right to their own beliefs and I do not judge anyone with beliefs different from mine. Neither do I apologize for the direction of my spiritual growth, which brought me to my current belief system.

At the time of John's death, through my study of *A Course in Miracles* as well as Dr. Caroline Myss' books *Sacred Contracts* and *Anatomy of the Spirit*, I had embraced the belief that we do not live just once. I also came to believe that prior to birth we determine what elements will be present in our lives, and what we choose to learn before we come to a life. We do this in collaboration with God, our guides and our angels. Given my new belief, I reasoned that I was the writer, producer, director, casting director and star of my own current life production. I believe John and Gary did the same with this life and we had our reasons on the other side for creating our intersecting experiences of this life. I hope to know those reasons in complete detail when I cross back over.

I came to understand how silly it was to be mad with God, and to scream at Him as I did repeatedly over the years after John's accident. John, Gary, our guides, our angels and I actually worked in consultation with Him to construct the "script" for this life. When we are told the biggest lesson we ever learn is to take responsibility for everything that happens to us I believe this is what that truth means. We helped create everything, so of course we are responsible. Part of our reason for being here is to learn specific lessons in order to reach ever-higher levels of spiritual understanding and growth. Those lessons are not God's punishment, for He does not punish. He loves us through all of the lessons we come to learn, no matter how we handle them. He has ensured that we are the masters of our fate. We are the creators of our lives, never the victims.

Prior to John's accident I embraced without question the belief system of the very conservative religion I grew up with. That religion had me believing that God is a vengeful, jealous God and one who judges and hands out punishment. Through my experience, and through searching for answers after the accident, I now reject that completely. I am now convinced it would be impossible for God to have such completely human emotions. He is a spirit without human limitations and, while He understands and forgives when we display them, it is impossible for Him to assume them.

From time to time some people who know my story have told me I've had bad luck. After considerable thought I came to completely reject that opinion. As a result of my experience with John, I do not for one moment believe that the Universe is so random as to be balanced on the whimsy of luck. Scientists tell us that the Universe is indeed balanced—right down to the smallest sub-atomic particle—and yet peacefully coexists and creates within a system of chaos as well. Astounding! Given that, how could the Universe function based on something as inequitable and ephemeral as luck?

I now believe what happens to us in our life is part of our plan, not the luck of the draw, and that we had specific reasons for creating such a plan. We came here to learn and our plan is therefore a guide to help us do just that. It is the only way my experience makes any sense to me. There is a reason why everything happens and it is part of our plan—the one we co-created. As I came to understand and believe this I also began to fully understand how our God-given free will functions. It is a huge part of the process of creating our life plan on the other side. It is equally important on this side because we are free to completely disregard the plan we designed. We are even free to disbelieve there is such a plan and to never spend one second trying to intuit what elements our plan may contain.

People who have been through life-altering experiences will often say that they are grateful for them because they learned so much, even though they would not want to repeat them. I now understand why people say that, and I couldn't agree more.

Those were my deepest thoughts as I learned of John's death and tried to process it. I was finally able to see the exquisite though painful tapestry our three lives had woven up to that point. I could see with clarity what we had all three learned as we worked our way through the whole shattering experience.

After being told of John's death, I called Gary, who was by then in school in Florida. I don't think he was any more surprised at the news than I was. We both felt that we should go to Las Cruces to settle John's affairs and dispose of his property. Neither one of us was looking forward to the experience but we wanted to do this one last thing for him as an act of love and closure. We knew John wanted to be cremated. Since Gary's schedule was such that he could not go with me until his spring break we decided to arrange for John to be cremated and his ashes stored until we got there in mid-March.

John and I had talked about death several times prior to his accident, and what we wanted done with our bodies. He was not a religious man, but he did believe in God and his concept of Heaven and Hell reflected his Methodist upbringing, but he had a decided spiritual aspect to him that he tried to keep under cover. Remember he had been a Marine, and being tough was what he was taught and lived. However, he showed that soft side to me during some of our deeper discussions of life and what it all means. In the early years of our marriage he used to tease me about my traditional beliefs, which reflected my conservative religious upbringing. He respected my beliefs, but he teased me anyway. He also watched me move from my dogmatic view of life to one of understanding and accepting that life isn't quite as black and white as we are often taught but instead has plenty of grays. John commented more than once that he liked my attempt to see life and others in a less judgmental way.

We often laughed about letting the other one know we'd made it when one of us crossed over. He used to say he would contact me from Hell because that was likely where he would be. (Little did we know he would encounter Hell right here on this Earth.) So I was shaken the day after he died to catch the unmistakable smell of cigarette smoke in my new home. John had always been a heavy smoker, and was up to four packs a day by the time of his death, in fact, it is very likely that's what caused his fatal heart attack. I hated his smoking and we often had words over his failure to quit. I am not a smoker and hadn't permitted anyone to smoke in my new home. So, at first I ignored the smell, thinking my imagination was getting the best of me, but it didn't go away and the longer I tried to ignore it the stronger it got.

I finally got up and went outdoors to see if maybe there was someone smoking outside the house. I lived in the middle of 13 wooded acres so it couldn't have been a neighbor. It also wasn't time for the man who cleaned my pool, or the one who mowed the lawn, to be at the house. They were both smokers but hadn't been there for a week or so. After a thorough search outside I found no one. I then searched each room of the house. Silly, I know, because I lived alone with two cats so unless one of them had taken up the habit the smoke was not coming from inside. For two days the smell of cigarette smoke stayed in that house. Then it was gone as suddenly as it had arrived. I believe to this day it was John letting me know he was gone—in the one unmistakable way he knew I would recognize.

Gary set in motion what we needed to get John's estate taken care of before we got to Las Cruces so our limited time there could be used efficiently. It seemed that March came quickly. Gary flew from Florida to my home in Alabama and together we flew to El Paso, Texas where we rented a car and drove on to Las Cruces. It was a long drive, with both of us quietly thoughtful, and late that evening before we pulled into our motel.

The next morning we made our way to the RV Park and on to John's trailer. We had no idea what to expect but there was no way we were prepared for what we encountered there. The window shades had been pulled down and his RV had been locked up by the sheriff after John's death in January and not opened until our arrival some two months later. The overpowering smell of stale cigarettes was the first thing to hit us. We both stepped back with our hands over our noses. After a few minutes, and armed with cleaning equipment, we forged into the trailer.

Gary began by opening windows to let in sunshine and air. The cigarette smoke was so heavy it was like walking through a fog that filled the trailer. We soon realized there was another smell—that made us gag. John must have been sick before he died, as there was dried vomit everywhere in the kitchen sink, bathroom and the bedroom. We didn't know it then but the virus that had made him sick had also been locked up in that trailer for two months and was still virulent.

John's clothes were strewn everywhere across the couch, on the bed and falling out of the closet. His beautiful suits, which he had worn proudly to the bank every day before his accident, were very much worse for wear, and I found that hard to take. I could only stay in the trailer for about 20 minutes at a time and would go outside to get a breath of fresh air. It was physically grueling but it was a bigger emotional toll, and one that hit me sooner than it hit Gary.

He was completely focused on getting the trailer cleaned and in the best shape possible before we put it on a consignment lot.

John's clothes went to a neighbor in the RV spot just across from his. He was a Vietnam vet who had never adjusted to civilian life—a nice man, but very fragile. He'd come back home with the same ghosts and nightmares that so many of his fellow Vietnam vets had. He told us John talked about Gary and me all of the time and was proud of both of us. As I'd suspected, John had taken our large album of family pictures with him when he left Alabama and proudly shown it to his neighbor as he talked about his former life.

We also needed to get John's truck ready to sell. Gary and I approached it with trepidation, not knowing how we would react to finally seeing the vehicle where John had tried so desperately to take his life. We'd been told there was a hole in the roof of the truck where the bullet exited but we knew seeing it would take the emotional impact to a whole new level. And it did. We were both very quiet as Gary opened the door. He looked up and put his finger on the hole in the interior roof of the truck. "Mom," he said, his voice hushed, "this is where the bullet went through the top of the truck after it went through Dad's head."

I could hardly see it through my tears as I finally came face-to-face with John's darkest hour. That wasn't the worst. Gary opened the glove compartment, prepared to clean it out. He pulled out a plastic bag and we both looked with horror at John's teeth. We knew the bullet had knocked out his teeth, but we weren't prepared to hold the proof in our hands. We have no idea why he saved those teeth, but we do know that there is a kind of pain that defies description. Seeing those teeth triggered that kind of pain.

By the end of the day, Gary and I were both physically and emotionally exhausted and dragged ourselves back to the motel. There we made plans to pick up John's ashes the next day. We both knew that John's wish had been to have his ashes scattered in Big Bend National Park in Texas. However, I was already starting to feel sick and Gary wasn't feeling well either. "Big Bend is a hard eight-hour drive away, Mom," he said. "Neither of us feels good, so Dad will just have to get along without Big Bend. Do you know anywhere closer that he might like?" I knew the perfect second choice.

When John was a banker in Houston he had a customer who used to loan us his vacation home in Ruidoso, New Mexico. We would trailer our horses over and ride in the beautiful mountains. Some of the best times we had together were there. I felt John would like having his ashes scattered in a place with such good memories so we made plans for the two-hour drive the next day.

Morning came and we set out from the motel to pick up John's ashes. It was yet another painful journey. We were shown into a waiting area at the Crematorium. It was very quiet. Then a man appeared and asked our names. We told him we were there to pick up John Nicholson's ashes. "Yes, we have them stored in a closet," he said. "Let me just get them."

At certain times, when an experience is so sad and overwhelming, you just have to resort to gallows humor to cope, so I said, "Gary, if your father knew he had been put on a shelf in a closet for two months he would have a fit!" When the man reappeared with John's ashes we had to work hard to keep our laughter to ourselves. On the way out Gary asked, "Mom, where shall I put him?" Again we resorted to gallows humor to survive. I told Gary to decide. "Well, Mom, I'm just going to throw him in the trunk." That started us laughing again. Of course, there was absolutely *nothing* funny about this situation but it was all just too overwhelming.

As we turned the car north to Ruidoso I was feeling just awful. About an hour out, I had to stop the car and throw up on the side of the road. John's virus had well and truly latched on to me. Gary took over driving duties and we had to stop a couple more times for me to throw up before I finally located the spot where I remembered John and I resting our horses. It is a place with a breathtaking view of the mountains and feels like you are on the top of the world. I knew he would like it and felt that he was somehow with us.

We got out of the car and stood on the spot I had chosen. I had prepared a short eulogy before I left home with the intention of reading it as we scattered his ashes in Big Bend. Not only were we not in Big Bend but I was also so sick I couldn't read the eulogy. Gary said he would read it as he slowly opened the container of ashes. I remember that it was almost eerily quiet and I could hear the wind blowing gently through the tall trees. We each reverently took handfuls of John's ashes. As Gary read the eulogy we both scattered them and, with the help of the wind, they were blown high into the magnificent blue sky. John was finally free.

JOHN'S EULOGY

Dear John,

As Gary and I stand here to free your ashes in Big Bend National Park as you requested, it is with many mixed emotions. I feel a bone-deep sorrow that your last thirteen years on this earth were lived within a devastating mental illness made worse by your lack of acceptance of your condition. It is that mental illness which separated you from your real self and from us. Your loneliness of soul grieves my heart. That you left us without anyone by your side is difficult to bear.

Though you thought otherwise, we loved you even when we could no longer live with you. I choose today to celebrate the many wonderful memories of our life together before the accident that took the real you from us and changed all of our lives forever. I choose to remember the day I called you at the bank after I had visited with my doctor to tell you that we were going to have a baby after almost giving up. You were ecstatic and said you knew we would have a son—and you were right.

I choose to remember your joy on family vacations to your favorite state, Colorado. I choose to remember the fun we had together with our horses whether riding or just hanging out with them at the barn. I choose to remember how proud you were of Gary, but how difficult it was for you to tell him that.

191

I choose to remember your delightful sense of humor and your awesome intellect. I choose to remember the man, the husband, who was my best friend.

My greatest hope is that you have found the peace, which escaped you the last years of your life. My greatest wish is that your new journey will bring you wisdom, love and an understanding of the events of this life you have just left.

Godspeed,
Donna

AFTERWORD

The ride from Ruidoso back to Las Cruces was a quiet one as neither my son Gary nor I felt well, emotionally or physically. For me it was also a ride through thirty years of memories. Reflecting on my life with John made me happy and sad at the same time. He was really gone—and that sank in as it never had before. During that ride I began to feel the gigantic hole his absence created for me in a much more intense way.

The finality of his death meant that the terrible sorrow I felt when I thought about his life and the damage the illness had done to all of us was reduced to an aching emptiness. I remembered the many times in the first two years after our divorce when I would abruptly wake up at night crying because I was dreaming that I was still married to John and continuing to experience the hideous aftermath of his accident. The immense relief and gratitude I felt when I realized it was only a bad dream was overwhelming. His death also made the treasured memories of the good times come alive. I could almost hear his laughter and see his face when he was teasing me, as he did so frequently prior to his accident. It was then that I realized I could no longer remember what his voice sounded like. That's when I knew he was gone for good from my life.

The journey that was my life from my marriage to John Nicholson in November of 1968, through our divorce in September of 1998, to his death in January 2004 was both the best and worst times of my life. Today I am grateful for the experience. It took me a very long time, diligent seeking and much study to finally understand why and for what purpose Gary, John and I suffered so greatly. Through this experience I've embraced a belief system which has produced the greatest spiritual growth I have had in my life. My belief system helps me understand that it is the way we see our problems, together with our attachment to specific solutions to those problems, which generates so much of what we call suffering on this Earth.

As a child I sang the Sunday School song "Let Go and Let God" which I realize now is all about surrender and acceptance which, through faith, generates our highest good. No need then to be attached to the outcome—it will be taken care of. Would I have ever asked for John to have such a life-alerting accident or such an insidious mental illness? Certainly not from an earthly perspective. Only from a spiritual perspective does it make any sense. From a spiritual perspective it answers my plea of "Why?" which I made to God repeatedly after John's accident. My new belief permits me to accept that John, Gary and I planned this accident and the aftermath before we incarnated to provide a context for all three of us to learn some of the lessons we came to this life to learn.

I believe the lessons on my path are balance, emotional independence and spiritual growth. Balance implies staying centered no matter what is going on around you. What I lived through with this experience most assuredly brought me great opportunity to acquire and practice balance. I know I have grown in this area because I have been able to keep my bearings along the way. After the accident I learned to cope with all I was presented with. Though it was extremely challenging, I grew in my confidence and ability to count on my emotional independence. I now believe that once the accident happened I became completely responsible for how I handled it. I count my spiritual growth through this experience as my ultimate area of growth.

Once I knew of John's unfaithfulness, I had to begin the journey to forgiveness as part of accepting responsibility for my reactions.

I struggled with it for such a long time. I have now finally reached forgiveness, which is the more important issue. I can honestly say I have come to the place where I bear no ill will toward John. I no longer struggle with the hurt, but instead I choose to remember the wonderful times we had together, the genuine love between us and the son we produced as a tribute to our relationship.

I am grateful I did not choose the path of bitterness, unforgiveness, blame and lack of acceptance. I certainly had that choice—and it was tempting. I did suffer but I realized that suffering looked at through the lens of my new belief system totally reframed the accident and its aftermath, which finally brought me to acceptance and peace. I now understand it. I now know the answer to "Why?" That understanding came at exactly the right moment. It came at the moment when I could finally accept it.

I also understand and accept that we are responsible for everything that happens to us. When I was first faced with that idea it offered a very bitter pill for me to swallow. Some people can't accept it at all. However, once accepted it gave me the clarity I was striving for. We are responsible for growing through our problems because, prior to our birth, we designed and placed them in our lives. Our problems are part of a grander design to provide a context for our growth. That's why they arrive on our doorstep throughout our life. There is always a reason why everything happens.

I am not the same person because of this experience. I know as I never knew before that I am capable of not only surviving great trauma and almost unbearable hurt and betrayal but I am also capable of growing because of it. Steel is tempered by fire. I went through the fire, stumbled and was scarred, yet came out whole on the other side. That is worth knowing.

Not only did I come through this trial by fire, but I also emerged with the wisdom that comes from making significant progress toward learning life lessons. I could never have gained such wisdom without such a trial, and just knowing that finally helped me accept what had happened to my husband. Learning those lessons put me on a higher spiritual path and has permitted me to use my experiences to extend love, compassion and understanding to others in need. As I began to take a more in depth look at what this tragic event in my life had taught me I realized what I had learned was not only humbling but also stunning in its scope. The life lessons I walked away with have helped me in so many ways. I now understand that:

✔ Guilt is a useless and destructive emotion. It should be treated as if it were poison because that is what it is. I spent so many years suffering needlessly from the effects of guilt. However, guilt is a very human reaction to pain as well as the feeling of powerlessness it fosters, and is often a destructive cornerstone of a relationship. For someone who has always been an overachiever (as I am), guilt is almost always the result when you see yourself as a failure. I thought I deserved my guilt because I had fallen short of my own standard of performance: I couldn't fix my husband. Had I been able to gain a perspective outside my relationship with John and his mental illness, I would have been kinder and gentler with myself. I would also have been far less judgmental of my actions.

I would never have treated my best friend or even my worst enemy with the disrespect I treated myself with during that time in my life, when I just kept heaping the guilt on and trying to carry my unnecessary burden. Had I been able to find some perspective, I would have been able to see that what I was doing in response to John's mental illness was the best I could at that moment, and that was not only good enough but in some cases it was extraordinary.

I have since forbidden guilt to cross my personal threshold, and I no longer beat myself up with it. I have also come to understand that guilt is not the same thing as sorrow and remorse, which are a normal part of any devastating experience. Guilt is in a class of its own, and has not one redeeming attribute.

✓ Even though I tried to handle the crisis in my life alone I should have realized sooner that was not possible. I had many people around me who were willing to help during my time of need. From the very beginning I should have just let them, with a grateful heart. I didn't have to learn that the hard way but unfortunately that's what happened.

✓ Crying is an act of cleansing and surrender. Surrender is critical to healing. I regret fighting it. I should have just let go. It is amazing how the act of surrender provides comfort, and very often just the right solution comes with it at just the right time. I fought surrender with all of my might as I dealt with John's mental illness because at the time it felt like a weakness I was not about to indulge. My suffering would have been so much less if I had learned the lesson of surrender sooner.

✓ How we deal with tragedy as well as life's trials and tribulations says a great deal about us. My experience reminded me that what happens to us is not as critical as what we do with it. I am so grateful that I ultimately used my dark night of the soul experience to pursue growth. I have used what I learned to help others as the opportunity has crossed my path. Although I was tempted to do otherwise at times, in the end I rejected bitterness, blame and an unforgiving heart. In rejecting that road I took the road less traveled. I'm thankful I did. As the poet Robert Frost predicted, that has made all the difference for me.

✔ None of us is ever alone—not ever. I was able to come to an understanding that what we can see and hear in this earthly dimension is not all there is—not by a long shot. There are always angels and guides by our side even if our earthly eyes cannot see them. They are always working for our greatest good. Sometimes acceptance of that spiritual truth was all that stood between me and being able to go on another day.

✔ There is always a reason why seemingly bad things happen. I had to finally get to a place where I could actively seek to understand that reason. I discovered that if the reason wasn't immediately clear to me then I just needed to strive for acceptance and the lesson to be learned. When my life was falling to pieces and I felt as if I would never find peace again I leaned on the idea Dr. Stephen Covey and people of wisdom through the ages have tried to instill in all of us—there are things we can control, and there are also things that we cannot. At the point of my greatest struggle with John's mental illness my school district sent me to be trained by Dr. Covey.

One of the most critical elements he taught me was that the events that are causing discord in your life are either in the circle of things you can control or in the circle of things you can only be concerned about, and perhaps exert some influence over, but which cannot be controlled. Once I became adept at knowing which events in my life belonged in the circle of concern and influence then I began the journey toward clarity, acceptance and peace.

✔ Humor is such a gift. Though at the time it seemed like a paradox for me to ever find humor within the devastating events of my life, when I did it lightened my load immensely. In the very thick of things, when it looked to me as if I would never laugh again, I remember telling a friend that I felt like my guardian angel had fallen in a hole and they had built a shopping center over her. When she started to laugh that gave me just the opportunity I needed, and we ended up laughing together until we cried. It was a refreshing oasis in the middle of my misery.

✓ Happiness is an inside job. I finally reached the point where I realized happiness did not emanate from somewhere outside of me. When I began to realize this truth, my first thought was it seemed illogical and counterintuitive. That's because my concept of happiness at the time was one of having everything working in my life, feeling care free and unobstructed with life's problems. I had always connected events, things, situations and even certain people with my happiness, or lack thereof.

I have since learned that my definition of happiness was very superficial. My lack of happiness was initially a great receptacle for my blame because I believed it came from somewhere other than me. When I finally understood that happiness is the result of my own decision-making, it became one of the most powerful and freeing beliefs I have acquired. I only wish I had been able to accept this during my struggles with John's mental illness.

✓ Security is an illusion. I learned in an instant that the world as you have known and loved it can be gone in the blink of an eye. That insight has taught me to appreciate and be sincerely grateful for the moment in which I am living.

Today I am blessed to continue working on behalf of children, which is a mission I came to this life with. I have never re-married. If I look deeply into my heart and become very honest with myself I know why. Marrying would take a level of courage to trust again that I am not sure I possess. Trust is the one unhealed area for me and, though I am still working diligently on it, I may run out of time before I experience healing in this life. Or perhaps I still have something to learn from my experience with John Nicholson before I am truly free. In either case, I can say with certainty that I have not yet encountered anyone as intelligent, humorous or able to go toe-to-toe with me as he was. He was a force to reckon with and, even though he was flawed as we all are, I must admit he left a huge hole in my heart and my life. However, I am clear that the greatest tribute to our relationship is our son who is a wonderful human being. His father would be so proud of him. I am now owned by two rescue cats and live alone in my adopted state of Texas in the beautiful Hill Country outside Austin. I live in gratitude for the peace and healing I have found after so many years of turmoil and uncertainty.

Though the memory of all I experienced and my ultimate loss can still produce tears, I have now come to peace and healing, which is what I asked for so long ago. There has been calm around the bend, as those long ago minnows taught me.

Final Thoughts

My last words are for those of you who are dealing with mental illness or who are in a relationship of family, marriage or parenting where there is mental illness of any kind, but particularly bipolar disorder and traumatic brain injury. Bipolar is a very pervasive condition. It is the world's sixth leading cause of disability. It is estimated that somewhere between five to ten million people in the United States alone have been diagnosed with this disorder and 30 million worldwide. No one knows how many more there are who have not presented themselves for diagnosis, either because they are ashamed and afraid of the stigma, which attaches to anyone with a mental illness, or because a bipolar disordered person very often lacks the insight to see themselves as mentally ill.

Some sources report that 1% of those with the disorder kill themselves. Yet others report that between 80–85% kill themselves, while others note percentages that lie between these two extremes. However, what is true and almost all sources support is that bipolar disorder creates a great proclivity for suicide and an unacceptable number of people who kill themselves.

Yet, even in the face of these startling facts they have yet to be met with an all out push to find a cure for bipolar disorder. (Experts are divided on whether it can be cured.) Or, if no cure, then at the very least a better way of managing it, and most certainly a more humane way of dealing with those who must be committed to a mental hospital. We should all be asking with one voice: WHY NOT?

Rather than support, in the past several years funding for treatment of mental illness has been substantially reduced. Where once there were at least a half million beds available in psychiatric hospitals there are now less than 50,000. It is also estimated that some 70,000 people diagnosed with mental illness are violent.

We have treated mental illness for so long, too long, as if it talking about it will somehow make it contagious. Out of shame we have kept it hidden. Hopefully, there is a new wind blowing, helping shift from shame to understanding that mental illness is a legitimate condition worthy of our best efforts to cure if possible, to discuss openly and compassionately, and to offer support for.

There is now an abundance of information on the Internet about bipolar disorder, as well as mental illness in general. There are also more personal stories about mental illness available online than ever before. However, it is still not accepted in our society as other illnesses are—but it can be if all of us who believe it should be speak with loud voices. Some celebrities have recently stepped up to raise their voices, speaking of their own experiences with bipolar disorder. But what of the rest of us? This book is my attempt—on behalf of my family—to be one of those voices.

I encourage others to find their voice and join me by telling their story. Let's create a critical mass with which to create more focused attention, and to provide understanding, support and comfort to the many people suffering from mental illness or supporting someone who is. If we work together, we can create the necessary pressure to demand the funding necessary for more and better research.

I also encourage those dealing with bipolar disorder or supporting someone who is to read Dr. Kay Redfield Jamison's book, *An Unquiet Mind*. It provided enormous understanding and comfort for both Gary and me. Since the publication of Dr. Jamison's book in 1995 another one has been written that is equally enlightening and helpful—*I Am Not Sick I Don't Need Help!* by Dr. Xavier Amador. Both books are trailblazers in the world of bipolar disorder.

In the appendices of this book I have provided a more complete bibliography of helpful books and links to websites. They did not exist for us in our time of need but they do for you. You will also find in the appendices answers to frequently asked questions about bipolar disorder, which include information on promising new medicines to manage it, new research that may provide a cure for bipolar disorder, plus information about traumatic brain injury. I have also included a simple template for those of you who are willing to share with me your own experiences with mental illness. I believe you will find the support you need in this section of the book. Seek and use that support.

Please remember above all else you are not alone. Many are on the same path you are on, and many of us have moved on to find our way to renewed joy and faith. You can too. My personal hope and prayer for you is that you will be given the strength and understanding to find your way to peace and healing.

May God bless and keep you.
Austin, Texas
March 2013

ACKNOWLEDGEMENTS

Shattered has been a long time in the making. It was necessary for me to first travel the road to peace and healing and then actually arrive there before I was able to write this story. Along the way and across many years people listened to my telling of the story. Without exception they said, "Donna, you must share this story. It will help so many people."

It was never that I doubted I would reach the point emotionally where I could write the story. That was not my concern. I was concerned because I did not believe I had the writing skills to do it justice. I am an avid reader—always have been—and I knew that, in order to really engage potential readers and provide help to others, I would have to find a way that I had never found before to write this true story. In the first week of January 2011 I did that.

I sat down in front of my computer that evening expecting to struggle, delete, rethink, rewrite and experience aggravating frustration. That did not happen. What did happen as I began to type was that an unmistakable presence entered my home office. I could not see it, but it was so real I turned around several times expecting to see someone. But there was no one. Then I began to write and the portion in this book titled "November 1999" describing John's attempt at suicide just poured out. I was astounded. That was the flow throughout the writing of this book.

So I must first acknowledge those unseen hands. Without the unseen guidance I do not know if *Shattered* would have become a reality. I am so grateful to whoever guided me, and any good that this book accomplishes is a tribute to the unseen help I consistently received

My son's assistance in collaborating with me and contributing his own perspective (see appendix A) has been instrumental in accurately telling our story. He helped me remember details I either had not known or had forgotten, bringing the book greater depth. He also created a chronological timeline of events after John's accident; researched names, locations and time periods and interviewed people from the past associated with John for detail as well as accuracy. His advice on marketing as well as his creation of the *Shattered* blog and website contributed immeasurably. Thank you so much, Gary.

Finding the right editor to work with me was quite a journey and again points to unseen hands. In April of 2011 I selected an editor in another state based on a recommendation, and it almost caused me to abandon this book. The comments on the manuscript were riddled with criticism delivered in a ridiculing manner and generally anything but encouraging. Going into the editing process, I had no confidence in myself as a writer. This confirmed it. Feeling very inadequate, I put the manuscript in a box, slammed the lid and threw it in the back of my office closet intending never to open it again.

The next day when a dear friend, Brittany Perkins, asked how the editing was going I told her that I apparently wasn't a writer after all, so I was through. She tried to reason with me, saying this isn't the only editor in the world and to get someone else, but I had lost heart. In retrospect I realize this was just part of timing being everything. I think I was still not quite ready to believe in *Shattered* as a reality. So now I am grateful to my first editor, and understand that person was a necessary part of my path to the creation of this book.

In early December of 2011 I started experiencing a niggling in the back of my mind to get the manuscript out of the box and give it another go. The niggling just would not stop. In the last week of December I felt moved to have a conversation about it with God. I said, "If I'm supposed to write this story then you have to send me the right editor because I do not have a clue where to find that person."

Two weeks later my friend Brittany called, saying, "You aren't going to believe this but I was just reading an article in Austin Woman Magazine written by a local writer. At the end of the article she provided her contact information, and she does editing and ghostwriting." At this point I was certain I needed a ghostwriter if this story was going to ever get written. So I excitedly and hopefully emailed the writer to ask if we could talk. I also attached the "November 1999" section and the introduction of *Shattered* so she could begin to get a sense of the book.

Given my earlier experience, I was expecting to either not hear anything from her or have her email me back saying, "Seriously? Are you kidding?" She did neither of those things and Julie Tereshchuk entered my life—sent by those unseen hands. She assured me I most certainly did not need a ghostwriter but what I did need was a developmental editor. She told me I was indeed a writer and so began our editing journey in April of 2012. I have loved every minute of the editing process, not because Julie doesn't offer criticism but because she does it in her loving, humorous, very direct way delivered in her delightful British manner. She has added immeasurably to the depth and breadth of *Shattered*. It was Julie who first pushed me to dig deeper to retrieve those painful memories that would be most meaningful to the reader. Julie, you are the best and I am so grateful our paths crossed. As I plan to continue to write, I am sure we will work together on other projects. Looking forward to it! Thank you Brittany for providing this critical link.

Grateful cannot even begin to describe how I feel about the national group I put together in May of 2012 to act as my first readers. They became my guinea pigs, which I shortened to GPigs. As Julie and I edited the book section by section most of the GPigs read it one edited section at a time. They provided critical feedback and it was used to make the final version so much better. The GPigs reflect the mass audience for whom *Shattered* is meant. Their diversity was purposeful. Most of the GPigs are voracious readers and they are all critical readers who would not hesitate to tell me the worst if necessary. There are a few GPigs who would rather do anything but voluntarily read a book. They have been my most ardent and engaged critics.

To all of you GPigs I can only say you are intrepid souls for hanging in there with me for an entire year. My gratitude to you for the gift of your time to serve as first readers is immense. Many of you were among the very people who encouraged me to write this story in the first place and then continued to encourage me to dig deeper, even though you knew it would be painful for me. Several of you brought a unique perspective to the role of first reader as you knew my husband, John. My deepest thanks to all of you.

APPENDIX A

Interview with Gary Nicholson
February 22, 2013

QUESTION: Were you close to your father growing up?

ANSWER: Growing up with two very smart and driven parents was challenging. Expectations were high and my father ruled with an iron fist. I had always had a rebellious streak and when I became a teenager it was in full force. As much as my dad hated my rebellion, it always made him nostalgic for his own days of rebellion. So in effect many things I did were allowed to slide from time to time. As I got older and started high school, things really changed. He became more withdrawn and aloof toward me. Our relationship became one of smoke and mirrors.

Things were changing in him and he was drinking more and more. He became obsessively controlling to the point to where I completely distanced myself. I always admired my father for what he accomplished in his banking career and how we both helped each other learn how to operate a farm after much trial and error and neighborly help. We made a pretty good team.

Q: What was your reaction when you heard about his accident in Colorado? Did you blame him and feel that the accident was at least partly his own fault?

A: The first two trips they took were a breathtaking experience for my father and his friends. When he came back he'd be really excited and already talking about the next trip. My father was pretty adventurous and the next trip (their third one) they planned was in a more extreme and remote wilderness. Some of the trails are really narrow and rocky. You have to go slow. I really feel that all of the men trained hard for this trip. I also jumped in and helped condition the horses and test out the rigging and packings on our ranch. Everything was in order. I think part of the accident was my father's fault—he probably had a hangover from the night before and might have been overconfident. Knowing my father, he was probably charging ahead to get as far up the trail as quickly as possible.

Neither of the two men on the trip with my dad is willing to tell me what really happened that day. That is something of a mystery to me.

When I heard about the accident, I wasn't exactly aware of him hitting his head. I remember his ribs being broken and having pneumonia and bruises on his back and arms. When he got home he seemed different. It was hard to describe because he was so physically injured. His speech was impaired a little and some words would drag a little too long.

I remember I was busy during this time getting ready to move away. I was working two jobs to pay off my truck and save some money for my trip. After a few weeks my father was moving around pretty easily in the house. You could tell that the injuries had knocked the wind out of him literally and figuratively. We talked a lot and he was excited about my move. Then as time grew near for me to leave and with the death of his father, the previous June, he started to break apart emotionally.

Q: How did your feelings towards him change in the years after the accident? Did he ever acknowledge that he had bipolar disorder?

A: Well, he was a different man when he came back from the mountains, and slowly he became a complete stranger to me. He was impossible to be around for very long without him starting some sort of drama with my mother or me. I joined the military mainly to get away from him. Before that I started my first semester of college and every day I was subject to his negative conditioning. Telling me I was worthless and a loser and how I'd never amount to anything and why am I wasting his money to go to school? I made my mind up to join the Navy and promptly quit school. What a relief that was.

He never once admitted to having bipolar disorder. He did often blame the medicine for killing his creativity. He really felt that he was just being creative.

Q: Do you think your mother kept you fully informed about your father's condition and treatment in the years following the accident?

A: Not really. By this time my father had pushed me away and created a divide in our family. The last time I was home he was running around accusing me of things I didn't do like eating all of their food and how they were going to starve to death. None of it was true, of course, but you could tell he was spiraling out of control. He also yelled at my mother during that time. It was really bad. He was so angry over nothing. My mother was so scared she went and lay down in her bed. I sat next to her and she pointed to a drawer in her chest and said it contained instructions on her funeral arrangements. It was scary and tense that night.

He would go from happy to mad to sad in minutes. It was a bad time. Being in the military didn't allow for me to come home much. I decided against coming home at all after that. I just couldn't take it. It was always such a bad time with him now. I never was able to relax when I was there and instead stayed on guard, never sleeping much. I was always on the lookout for anything about to happen. I actually stayed with friends mostly when I was there in town just to create space, but then my father and I would fight because he demanded to know the address and phone numbers of my friends. I never gave in. I considered myself to be on my own now and I only took orders from my military chain of command

My father made it very hard to be in his life so I walked out and kept him at a distance leaving my mother behind too. I figured it was safer anyway for my mom if he felt less threatened with me around. He loved to call me and tell me how devastated my mother was that I wouldn't come home. I was not happy that my mom kept my father's first commitment from me. I did not know until I had come home for Thanksgiving. It was all so shocking that I didn't really have time to feel anger. I was trying to grasp the situation that was happening around me. My father seemed calm at first but he cycled through emotions quickly and we had to apprehend him once during the thanksgiving meal. It was so exhausting emotionally and physically.

Q: Talk about the day in February 1998 when your father pulled his gun on you and threatened to kill you. Have your feelings about it altered over the years?

A: Well, I had just come back from a six-month deployment and tour of duty in the Persian Gulf. It took me a while to come down to the civilian world level in terms of not having to be on high alert all of the time. It took me a year to fully shake it off. I would have dreams about alarms going off and wake up in a cold sweat thinking I'd missed a watch or duty assignment. I was so alert I swear I could smell the situation about to happen. I could feel something but I didn't know what. Every move, every interaction, everything I did that day with my dad seemed like a chess game. He had not seen me in a while and he felt threatened. I could feel it. As the day went on he became more agitated. When he finally snapped on my mother I went and stood between them and told him he better not lay a hand on her. I had never spoken to my father like this before, but given the situation brewing before me, I did what I had to do. When I yelled back at him to stop, he stopped immediately and with that he said, "I've got something that will take care of you." And walked past me to the bedroom. I knew what was next and in a split second I determined that removing myself from the situation was the best bet. After all, I was the threat. I ran next door and told the neighbor to call the cops. My heart pounded as I waited for the sound of a gun to go off. I wasn't sure if he would try and kill my mother or himself or both. Seconds seemed like hours waiting for the cops to get there. Luckily the station was only minutes away.

Q: How did you find out about your father's suicide attempt, and what were your reactions? How do you feel about it now?

A: I got a call from my mom who had just gotten a call from the neurosurgeon treating my dad and she told me what had happened. I was shocked. I remember my cousin was helping me figure out what to do next. Since my mom was divorced from him there was not anything she could do legally. That is not to say she was not helpful. She just didn't have any rights. Luckily she was paying his insurance so the insurance company paid most of the bills. We knew it would run out and he would have to start paying for care so we decided upon the VA center in Houston. I really don't think much about the suicide in the scheme of things. I remember more of the good times these days. We had many before the accident happened.

Q: After you learned of your father's suicide attempt, you flew there to be with him. What happened once you arrived?

A: Once I arrived in Albuquerque I went immediately to my hotel and then called the hospital to find out what area he was in. I then went to the hospital. Until she opened her mouth, I was unaware that the person at the front reception area was also the one who answered the phone when I called from the hotel. I found out later that she was tipping off my father's female friend that I was in the hospital. She made herself scarce for the next few days and I seemed to always miss her coming and going. Eventually she came by and tried to ease me into believing that she was there in my father's interest. She became very confrontational and threatened me with a lawyer.

Eventually the hospital got involved and we had a hearing to contest the validity of her power of attorney. They asked what I wanted to do with my father after his treatment. I responded that we wanted to take him to the VA assisted living and rehabilitation center in Houston and help him get back on his feet. Dad's girlfriend said that he wanted to go back to Arizona now that he was cleared of all charges against him. She also said we abandoned him and that my mom divorced him. She said we didn't care. I tried to retaliate by questioning her role against me as his actual family member. She was also wearing my grandmother's engagement ring and passing it off as a gift from her "fiancé", my dad. Her lawyer was also present but was told he was not allowed to speak at the hearing.

Nothing was resolved in that meeting other than they would let the courts decide and that it was out of their hands. We were all warned not to try and attempt to help him escape. The hospital director told dad's girlfriend that her lawyer was not allowed inside his room or on the floor he was on. She scoffed at this and proceeded to take him up to my father's room. I walked up there and asked him to leave. They were both busy trying to get my father to sign papers attesting to his ability to make his own decisions. My father lying in his bed was in and out of consciousness. I immediately called the director and he had the lawyer removed.

The director was not very effective in enforcing his rules and eventually he gave up and Dad's girlfriend was given full run of his everyday activities until one day a nurse discovered that she had unhooked my dad's IV. She was made to sign an agreement that she wouldn't touch anything. She somehow talked Dad into a power of attorney beforehand and somehow in the State of New Mexico a power of attorney trumps blood relative.

Q: How did you hear your father had died?

A: I was at a friend's house watching football. When I got home my roommate told me that my mother had called. I called her back and she told me. I had not seen or heard from my father in five years. I can't say I was sad at first. More shocked and relieved. I finally felt like I didn't have to look over my shoulder anymore.

Q: Describe the trip you and your mother made to Las Cruces after your father's death to dispose of his personal belongings.

A: When we got to Las Cruces we went straight to the hotel and being that it was late in the day we decided to start working on his trailer that next day. My father had a neighbor who I was able to get in touch with before I went out to Las Cruces. He and I talked many times before the trip. I always had a thousand questions for him. When we got settled into the hotel I decided to go see him. I tried to imagine my father's life here. It all seemed so foreign to me. A different life. A life I wasn't privy to. We focused on his trailer first before exploring the truck.

The trailer wasn't so much a mess as it was super dusty and the ceilings were tar-covered from the cigarette smoke. (He once called his RV a "prison" when he wrote a letter to my mother pleading for her to let him come back.) When I finally got to the truck to clean it out I opened up the glove box and inside was a Ziploc bag containing his teeth and bridge. I looked up at the top of the truck and saw the bullet hole. I ran my hand over it and then looked at it from the outside. No attempt was ever made to fix it. Probably because my father wouldn't acknowledge that he actually shot himself.

Q: What are your feelings towards your father today?

A: Once he died I had a hard time wrapping my head around it all. Eight months earlier my relationship with my girlfriend of three years ended and I also moved to California to attend film school during that time so it was a tough time for me in many ways. I forgave him finally about two year later. It's been many years now since he died.

Those two long days of cleaning up his effects just had both my mother and me shaking our heads and wondering why. While cleaning the truck out and seeing the bullet hole in the top of the truck, I sat back down in the cab and started it up. I remember sitting there and wondering what it was like that day in 1999 when he shot himself.

Bipolar Disorder & Traumatic Brain Injury

QUESTION: What is bipolar disorder?

ANSWER: Bipolar disorder is also known as manic depression. It is generally thought to be an imbalance of the chemicals in the brain that causes extreme mood swings between depression and manic behavior. These mood swings are not just the normal ups and downs most people experience. They are much more severe. This disorder is manifested in different ways in different people.

Bipolar I Disorder is the classic manic-depressive form of the illness and creates at least one manic episode and one depressive episode or a mixed episode.

Bipolar II Disorder manifests in episodes of hypomania and severe depression but doesn't result in full-blown manic episodes.

Cyclothymia is a milder form of bipolar disorder. It manifests in cyclical mood swings but the symptoms are less severe than full-blown mania or depression.

Q: What are the characteristics displayed by someone with bipolar disorder?

A: The symptoms vary widely and can manifest differently in people with the disorder. The **manic** phase presents feelings of heightened energy, creativity and euphoria. People in a manic episode talk rapidly, frequently interrupting their speech because their thoughts are coming so fast. They sleep very little and can go days without sleep. They are hyperactive, believe they are all powerful, invincible, destined for greatness, and are oblivious of any obstacles in their way. They believe that money is in inexhaustible supply therefore they can either spend or give away large sums of money while on the manic side of the disorder. They can be unusually high energy and optimistic or extremely irritable.

In a manic episode they tend to spiral out of control and behave recklessly: gambling away savings, engaging in inappropriate sexual activity, making foolish business investments and spending money recklessly. They can also become angry and aggressive—which causes them to pick fights, lashing out at everyone and blaming anyone who criticizes their behavior. Some people even become delusional and begin hearing voices.

Bipolar **depression** usually involves extreme irritability, guilt, unpredictable mood swings and feelings of restlessness. While in a depressive episode, people tend to move and speak slowly, sleep for long uninterrupted periods, display feelings of hopelessness, sadness and emptiness. They have memory loss, an inability to focus and feelings of worthlessness. The most dangerous feelings they experience during a depressive episode are their thoughts of death and a desire to kill themselves.

Mixed episodes of bipolar disorder are a combination of both mania or hypomania and depression symptoms. Common manifestations are depression combined with agitation, irritability, anxiety, insomnia, distractibility and racing thoughts. It is this combination of high energy and low mood that creates the high risk for suicide. Both the signs of depression and mania can often be seen in a mixed episode lasting as little as an hour.

Mixed bipolar disorder is common with people diagnosed with bipolar disorder. It is estimated that 20-70% of people with bipolar experience mixed episodes. Some researchers think that people who develop bipolar at a younger age, particularly in adolescence, may be more likely to have mixed bipolar disorder.

Q: Is bipolar disorder inherited and what exactly causes it?

A: Researchers and doctors are somewhat divided over the exact causes of bipolar disorder. Most agree that it has no single cause but there seem to be certain people who are genetically predisposed to bipolar disorder. However, not everyone with an inherited potential develops the illness indicating that genes are not the only culprits. Some brain imaging studies indicate physical changes in the brains of people with bipolar disorder.

Other research studies show neurotransmitter imbalances, abnormal thyroid function, circadian rhythm disturbances and high levels of the stress hormone cortisol as a cause of bipolar disorder. Even external factors in the environment and psychological makeup are thought to act as triggers that can set off or worsen new episodes of mania or depression. Some studies indicate that a severe trauma or extreme stress can trigger the disorder.

The National Institute for Mental Health (NIMH) believes it is an inherited disease. More than two-thirds of people with bipolar disorder have at least one close relative with the illness or with unipolar major depression.

Statistics on inheriting the disease vary widely. One source (see Source 7 below) reports that when one parent is affected, the risk to each child is 15–30%. When both parents have the disorder the risk increases to 50–75%. There is some research that indicates it can also skip a generation.

There is a diagnosis gap for this disease. Only one in four people receive an accurate diagnosis over a three-year period. Research has shown that many people with this disorder suffer as long as 10 years with the symptoms before receiving an accurate diagnosis. Dr. Wes Burgess, in his book *Bipolar Handbook*, reports that almost 70% of bipolar patients had been misdiagnosed more than three times before receiving their correct diagnosis. Bipolar disorder is difficult to diagnose because it can mimic other conditions, such as attention deficit hyperactivity disorder (ADHD).

Q: At what age do most people with bipolar disorder manifest the symptoms?

A: The median age of onset is 25 years but it can begin in childhood and often doesn't appear until a person is in their 40's or 50's.

Q: Is there any difference between men and women, races, ethnicities or socio-economic backgrounds when it comes to having bipolar disorder?

A: Bipolar apparently affects all races, ethnic groups and socio-economic backgrounds. However, some researchers have found that, while there is no difference in the rate at which men and women have bipolar disorder, there may be a difference in how it develops. These researchers report that women are three times more likely to experience rapidly cycling bipolar, i.e. cycling from depression to mania to depression or mania to depression to mania. According to this research, women have more depressive episodes and more mixed episodes than men. (*Journal of Clinical Psychiatry*, 1995.) It is also thought that female hormones and reproductive factors may influence bipolar disorder as well as its treatment.

One study indicates that the late onset of bipolar disorder can be associated with menopause. Researchers reported that among women with the disorder almost one in five reported severe emotional disturbances during the onset of menopause. Studies have also looked at the link between bipolar disorder and premenstrual symptoms. The results suggest that women with mood disorders, including bipolar disorder, have more severe symptoms of PMS. The most compelling evidence of this link is found during pregnancy and the postpartum period. Women with bipolar disorder who are pregnant or have recently given birth are seven times more likely than other women to be admitted to the hospital for their bipolar disorder and twice as likely to have a recurrence of symptoms. (See Source 4, below.)

Q: At what rate do people with bipolar disorder attempt and/or commit suicide?

A: Due to the high incidence of incorrect or delayed diagnosis bipolar often accounts for 9.2 years of reduction in the expected life span. Within that number lays the statistic that up to 1 in 5 bipolar disordered people complete suicide. However, the statistics on suicide and bipolar disorder are hard to nail down and have wide variation making it difficult to have any confidence in the data. For example, in his book, Dr. Burgess reports that 30% of individuals with bipolar will attempt suicide during their lives and 20% will succeed. Yet other sources report both lower and higher incidences of attempted suicide and suicide. What is known and what we can put confidence in is the fact that suicide is more common in bipolar depression than in unipolar depression, panic disorder or even schizophrenia; and that when bipolar disorder is adequately treated the suicide rate goes down dramatically.

Q: Is there a relationship between physical health issues and bipolar disorder?

A: Yes. The February 2009 *Medical Journal of Psychiatric Services* published some startling information regarding bipolar and a range of medical conditions. It was found that bipolar disorder can double the risk of early death from a wide range of medical conditions, including many that can be controlled through diet and exercise.

Consider:

✔ 35% of people with bipolar are obese, which is the highest for any psychiatric illness

✔ People with bipolar are three times more likely to develop diabetes than someone in the general population.

✔ People with bipolar are 1.5-2 times more likely to die from conditions such as heart disease, diabetes and stroke.

✔ People with bipolar are at higher risk for substance abuse. Almost 60% abuse drugs or alcohol. Substance abuse is found especially in those with a more severe bipolar disorder as well as those who are not managing the disorder, or managing it poorly.

✔ Bipolar disorder affects energy level, appetite, sleep patterns and sex drive.

Q: Is bipolar a common mental illness?

A: The World Health Organization (WHO) reports that bipolar disorder is the world's sixth leading cause of disability. Statistics reported by the Depression and Bipolar Support Alliance (DBSA) indicate that approximately 5.7 million adult Americans or about 2.6% of the U.S. population age 18 and older are bipolar. Other sources place that figure between 5-10 million in the U.S. and approximately 30 million worldwide. Those figures are thought to be conservative estimates as bipolar disordered people are often misdiagnosed, do not present themselves for diagnoses, and/ or lack the insight to realize that they are experiencing symptoms of the disorder. In short, bipolar disorder is very pervasive.

Q: How is bipolar disorder treated?

A: Lithium is the most common drug used for the treatment of bipolar. Success rates for bipolar disorder treatment with lithium vary from highs of 70- 85% to lows of 40-50%. (Surgeon General Report for Mental Health, 1999.) Nearly 9 out of 10 people with bipolar disorder are satisfied with their treatment, although they report side effects remain a problem. Caution should be taken with this statistic because a large number of people diagnosed with bipolar disorder refuse to take their medicine precisely because of the side effects and refuse more often than not to participate in psychological counseling. They just don't talk to anyone about their issues unless it is someone supporting them, such as family members.

New treatments for bipolar disorder (see Source 6 below) are emerging because more people are being diagnosed. Even though lithium is the standard treatment, over 75% of those who take the drug report side effects. One exciting and promising treatment being studied is one that is typically used for seasickness—scopolamine, which has shown to improve overall mood, a change that can last from weeks to months. Scopolamine skin patches are now being used for the treatment of bipolar disorder with promising results.

Q: Is there a cure for bipolar disorder?

A: The medical community is divided on whether bipolar or related mental illnesses can be cured. Everyone concedes that bipolar has its roots in physiology, meaning it is the result of something physical not mental, but its symptoms manifest as mental issues. There are some encouraging research advances, which will at least make the treatment of this disorder much more effective and efficient, and which may lead to a cure in the distant future.

For over 10 years, the Heinz C. Prechter Bipolar Research Fund based at the University of Michigan Depression Center has been conducting cutting edge stem cell research aimed at unlocking the secrets of bipolar disorder. New stem cell lines from the skin of adults living with bipolar disorder are providing the researchers with an unprecedented opportunity to look in depth at the genetic and biological basis of this disorder. Scientists conducting the research link their findings—such as how gene expression is affected by different medications—to extensive clinical and demographic data from the cell donors who are participants in an ongoing, long-term study of hundreds of individuals with bipolar disorder.

Currently, the best treatments for bipolar disorder are only effective for 30-50% of patients, according to Dr. Melvin McInnis. Dr. McInnis tells us that new discoveries have been limited in the past partially due to the lack of access to tissue and cells from individuals with bipolar disorder. Due to the Prechter Fund research, and the advances in stem cell research, that is changing. We most often associate stem cells with therapies to treat diseases but this research application is a great example of using stem cells to study the mechanisms of disease, according to Dr. Sue O'Shea. Dr. O'Shea says this offers hope to those with bipolar disorder. Researchers do caution that new treatments resulting from this work could be a decade or more away.

New research is also being done to consider the link between DNA and bipolar disorder. DNA analysis is used to identify the wide variance in the way this disorder manifests itself in different people. From this research new treatments will very likely emerge.

However, until more research dollars are made available not only will we not be able to determine if bipolar can be cured, we will also not be able to find our way to better medication and treatment protocol.

Q: Can people with bipolar disorder live a normal life?
A: Yes. Many people with bipolar disorder enjoy successful careers, happy family lives and satisfying relationships. However, living with bipolar disorder is challenging and it must be strategically

managed. It requires long-term, consistent, closely monitored management. Medication alone is not enough. Studies have shown that combining psychotherapy with the appropriate medication in the appropriate dosage is the most effective treatment strategy. There are some specific strategies, which should be considered:

✓ Using **Family Focused Treatment** (FFT) in addition to appropriate medication was shown to produce significantly lower relapse to manifestation of the disorder (11%) than medication alone (61%) over a nine-month period.

✓ **Cognitive Behavioral Therapy** (CBT) in combination with the appropriate medication reduced depressive symptoms by 7.3% as opposed to a reduction of only 2.5% with medication alone in a 2001 study.

Q: What is Traumatic Brain Injury?

A: According to the Individuals with Disabilities Education Act of 2004 (IDEA), traumatic brain injury applies to open or closed head injuries resulting in impairments in one or more areas, such as cognition, language, memory, attention, reasoning, abstract thinking, judgment, problem solving, sensory, perceptual and motor abilities, psychological behavior, physical functions, information processing, and speech. Traumatic brain injury does not apply to brain injuries that are congenital or degenerative or to brain injuries induced by birth trauma (Sec. 300.8 (c) (12).

Q: How many people incur traumatic brain injury and can it result in death?

A: Annually 3.5 million people in the United States incur a traumatic brain injury. 50,000 people die due to a TBI each year. It is estimated that a brain injury occurs every 20 seconds in the

U.S. Traumatic brain injuries are more common in the U.S. than breast cancer, multiple sclerosis or spinal cord injury. (*Mindstorms*, John W. Cassidy M.D.)

Q: Have many service men and women who have been in combat incurred a traumatic brain injury?

A: Traumatic brain injury is considered the "signature injury" of the conflicts in Iraq and Afghanistan because increasingly soldiers are surviving nearby bomb blasts. These bomb blasts produce brain injury through pressure waves that "shake" the brain. If the injury is severe enough it can cause irreversible results including depression, anxiety, personality changes, aggression, acting out and social inappropriateness. (National Alliance on Mental Illness Veterans Resource Center.)

It is estimated that 350, 000 servicemen and women have to date come home from Iraq and Afghanistan with mild to severe brain injuries. Much of the advancement in the treatment of TBI is due to these wars and the veterans who require effective treatment for this type of wound.

Q: Does traumatic brain injury lead to bipolar disorder and other mental illnesses?

A: Mood disorders are more frequent after brain injury and both depressive and manic episodes are found with an increased risk of aggression. Bipolar is often considered a secondary result of traumatic brain injury and occurs in as many as 9% of persons with a TBI. Drugs typically used to treat bipolar disorder such as antipsychotic drugs may actually exacerbate the symptoms of bipolar (both the manic and depressive side of the disorder) when a TBI has occurred. Even though mood disturbances can occur with injury to either hemisphere of the brain, mania has been primarily associated with right-side frontal lobe injury.

Dr. Robert van Reekum's (Baycrest Centre for Geriatric Care) results from a comprehensive review of data from the

1990s joins a growing body of evidence that supports the fact that a TBI causes many psychiatric illnesses including bipolar disorder.

Sources:

1. Bipolar Disorder Secondary to Head Injury; A Medline Search by Ivan K. Goldberg, MD
2. National Alliance on Mental Illness
3. IDEA, 2004
4. WebMD.com, "Women With Bipolar Disorder," September 6, 2012
5. FoxNews.com, October 10, 2010
6. NewsMax.com, New Treatments for Bipolar Disorder, March 23, 2011
7. Bipolar-lives.com, Bipolar Disorder Statistics August 3, 2012
8. WebMD.com, "Mixed Bipolar Disorder," July 18, 2012
9. HelpGuide.org, "Understanding Bipolar Disorder, July 18, 2012
10. Blue Cross Blue Shield Association, "New Bipolar Disorder Treatments Tested," Malcolm Ritter, July 20, 2011
11. Baycrest News and Media Information, Toronto, Canada, July 18, 2012
12. VFWLady.com, "Traumatic brain Injuries in OIF/OEF: Record Number of Vets Seeking Mental Healthcare," October, 19, 2011
13. ABCNews.com, "Do People of All Ages Get Bipolar Disorder, And Does Bipolar Manifest Itself At Different Ages?" September 6, 2012

APPENDIX C

Support Organizations and Websites
Bipolar Disorder and Traumatic Brain Injury

National Alliance of Mental Illness (NAMI): 3803 N. Fairfax Dr., Ste 100, Arlington, VA 22203, 703-524-7600, www.nami.org

Depression and Biploar Support (DBSA): 730 N. Franklin St., Suite 501, Chicago, IL 60654-7225, 800-826-3632, www.dbsalliance.org

National Institute of Mental Health (NIMH): 6001 Executive Blvd. Room 6200, MSC 9663, Bethesda, MD 20892-9663, 866-615-6464, www.nimh.nih.gov

Bipolar Significant Others: www.bpso.org

Brain Injury Association of America (BIAA): 1608 Spring Hill N, Suite 110, Vienna, VA 22182, 703-761-0750, www.biausa.org

American Veterans with Brain Injuries: www.avbi.org

SERVICE FOR BRAIN INJURY (SBI)-: 60 Daggett Drive, San Jose,
CA 95134, 408-434-2277, www.sbicares.org

DEFENSE AND VETERANS BRAIN INJURY CENTER (DVBIC):
www.dvbic.org

WOUNDED WARRIOR PROJECT: 12672 Silicon Drive, Suite 105,
San Antonio, TX 78249, 210-569-0300,
www.WoundedWarriorProject.org

NOTE: These organizations are all nonprofits whose only mission is
to serve those with mental illness, traumatic brain injury or their
supporters. They exist financially either on memberships, donations
or both. When budgeting for your charitable giving, please keep
them in mind. All of these organizations are contributing greatly to
fostering the understanding of mental disease and TBI, supporting
efforts to provide healing to many and bringing comfort to families.

BIBLIOGRAPHY

A selected bibliography of books offering support for, and under-standing of, bipolar disorder and traumatic brain injury

Amador, Xavier & Johanson, Ana-Lisa. *I Am Not Sick. I Don't Need Help!* Vida Press, 2000, 2007, 2011.

Andreason, Nancy C. *Brave New Brain: Conquering Mental Illness in the Era of the Genome.* Oxford University Press, 2004.

Cassidy, John W. & Woodruff, Lee. *MindStorms.* DaCapo Press, 2009.

Eron, Judy. *What Goes Up: Surviving The Manic Episode of a Loved One.* Baracade Books, 2005.

Fast, Julie A. & Preston, John D. *Loving Someone With Bipolar Disorder.* New Harbinger Publications, second edition, 2012.

Jamison, Kay Redfield. *An Unquiet Mind.* Alfred A. Knopf, 1995.

Horan, Carol. *A Family's Secret: Bipolar Disorder on Treetop Lane.* CreateSpace Independent Publishing Platform, 2005, 2012.

Woodruff, Lee & Bob. *In An Instant: A Family's Journey of Love and Healing.* Random House Trade Paperbacks, 2008.

SHARE YOUR STORY

If you are willing to share your personal story of mental illness, traumatic brain injury, or your role as a supporter of someone with these conditions, please email DrDonna@shattered-book.com with the following information:

✔Your Name

✔Date of Submission

✔Details of Your Story (under 800 words, please)

✔Whether you are willing to permit me to share your story with others (with or without including your name)

Together, we can use our stories to further the cause of these critical illnesses.

Be sure to visit Donna Nicholson's website
www.shattered-book.com

for more information on mental illness and traumatic brain injury